The Boat

BOOKS BY TOM KELLY

Tenth Legion
Dealer's Choice
Better on a Rising Tide
The Season
The Boat

The Boat

Tom Kelly

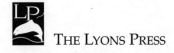

THE LYONS PRESS

Printed in the United States of America

10 9 8 7 6 5 4 3 2 1

Map illustrations by Michael Simon
Design by Sans Serif, Inc.
Library of Congress Cataloging-in-Publication Data

Kelly, Tom, 1927–
    The boat / Tom Kelly.
      p.   cm.
    ISBN 1-55821-640-5
    1. Boatbuilding. I. Title.
   VM321.K425   1998
   623.8'2023'092—dc21   97-22002
                                 CIP
"Key of H" has previously appeared in *Field & Stream*.

Contents

1

Origins

THERE ARE FEW PLACES on earth that lend themselves as readily to philosophical discussions as do duck blinds.

Even single-occupant blinds—where there is nobody else to talk to and you would expect a lack of conversation unless the sole inhabitant has a split personality and is prone to having double-identity discussions—have a tendency to become ruminative. They tend to encourage philosophical thought processes even if there is no one else there to have philosophical discussions with, which very frequently leads to walks down memory lane.

Like one morning last fall, for example.

To begin with, it wasn't so much a blind as it was a stand. Rather than sitting on anything, I was standing in knee-deep water next to the boat, alone. For seconds, the morning had been lively enough to keep a half-dozen occupants of a blind busy, let alone a sole proprietor.

The October hurricane—we had so many in 1995 the weather service almost ran out of names to call them—had blown down several thousand feet of water oak across that last slough running south toward Major's Creek. To compound the felony, the month of November, normally the driest month we have, dropped enough rain in the first four days to put the river at flood stage, believe it or not, the week before Thanksgiving. There is not supposed to be a flood in the river swamp the week before Thanksgiving. It says so, right here in the small print.

Such a volume of water, in direct contravention of the contract, coupled with the necessity to go to other places and salvage higher-value timber that the hurricanes had blown down, threw the area between the last slough and the north bank of Major's Creek into that category best defined as informed neglect.

It needed fixing, and under normal circumstances it would be corrected quickly. But with the situation as it was last fall, nobody was going to trouble himself for five minutes with blown-down water oak in eighteen inches of water.

Four-hundred-dollars-per-thousand pine sawlogs, blown flat across an area the size of half a county, turning blue while they waited for the advent of the southern pine beetle, eliminated any priority that defective water oak with epicormic branches may have had under normal circumstances.

As a consequence, getting a boat to the back side of the beaver pond that borders this last slough—in the dark, with everything looking different because so many of the marker trees had been blown down and were prostrate—was not only slow, it was glacial, and it was frustrating to boot.

Water oak cross-pollinates with both laurel oak and willow oak, so to be intellectually honest about it, you can't really call it water oak, although everybody does. The tree is a genetic mixture of all three in various proportions—a biological meat loaf, as it were—but all three of the partners in miscegenation have a single characteristic that breeds true in the resultant offspring: There is no depth to the root system at all.

I can quote no specific studies as to the depth of the root system of entire-leaved red oak, the name commonly used for the water/willow/laurel mixture, but it can't be much more than two feet.

All across the swamp, in the area of the blowdowns, there are circles of earth ten feet in diameter held upright like giant wheels by the boles of the blown-down tree protruding from the center of the circle. None of these wheels of earth, regardless of its diameter, is more than thirty inches thick.

By the time I had struggled around all the obstacles, after first deciding which blowdown constituted an obstacle, it was beginning to get light, and my arrival at the open part of the pond was about fifteen minutes later than it ought to have been.

A flock of a dozen or so mallards flushed out of the middle of the opening as I pushed out into it. I crossed over to the east side, pulled the pirogue under a couple of bushy cypress saplings, and standing in thigh-deep water next to the boat, untied the sack and began to throw the decoys out into the open water.

I read one time that Harry Houdini used to sit at a table and practice tying and untying knots in a piece of twine with his toes. He went through such an exercise to make all of his appendages limber, active, and useful so they could help remove the chains and ropes that tied him when he was dropped overboard—bound, chained, and nailed up in a packing crate—for one of his escape performances.

The article did not say what Houdini did with his hands while he was occupied in limbering up his toes. Wrote letters to his family probably, or practiced dealing seconds and thirds from a deck of cards for his poker sessions.

Houdini could probably keep his footing in thigh-deep water, hold the boat steady with one hand, use the other hand to uncase the gun and load it, take decoys out of the sack, untangle the weights, and throw them out into the water, watch for ducks, call at the proper time, and stay hidden—all simultaneously.

Whatever skill he may have eventually developed with his toes would not help him in this particular instance, because his toes would be encased in chest-high waders and buried a couple of inches deep in the mud throughout the operation.

He would be left with only the use of his hands, teeth, and elbows, but I am not for an instant saying that he could not have done it. He probably could have, and drunk a cup of coffee and whistled the violin solo from the overture to *Orpheus in the Underworld* at the same time.

But those of us who are substantially more disadvantaged in motor skill dexterity—those of us who in fact can barely pick up a piece of rope with our toes, let alone tie knots in twine with them—do a lot better when we get to the pond early enough to do several of these things at a far more deliberate pace. Say, like mostly one thing at a time.

About the only thing we of the slow set—those of us without limber toes who can't walk and chew gum at the same time—can do to help is to buy weighted-keel decoys.

Weighted-keel decoys (as opposed to water-keel decoys) allow you to do two things at one time. You can stand at the boat and throw the decoys as far as you are able, and they right themselves after they get there. It tends to be a little sloppy, and you generally end up with a few of them too close together, but when you get there late to begin with, and things are already beginning to happen before you arrive, it is a help to be able to load the gun, stand at the boat and keep yourself partially hidden, and still retain the ability to shoot while you set things up.

Sloppy or not, it beats the hell out of wandering around the pond with no gun, dragging a sack of decoys behind you, while early arrivals circle the incomplete stool wondering what in the world that thing is that's wading around among the lighted ducks.

There were enough arrivals after daylight for me to be able to shoot a pair of mallards who had gotten up a little late and then a pair of woodies who just happened to wander by.

While I was standing there waiting for the fifth duck, a drove of turkeys that had roosted partially on the modest bluffs at the foot of the pond and partially out in the swamp itself began to tree yelp to one another as they woke up. They were all young gobblers as far as I could tell, because as two of them left their trees up on the bluff and sailed out into the swamp to join the majority of the drove gathering out there, it looked as if half the length of each flying bird was neck.

After they got there, one of those early-morning arguments broke out. While there were probably no more than twelve or fifteen turkeys in all, they did a credible imitation of the amount of noise made by fifty.

When I shot the fifth duck, everybody out there shut up, but only for a minute or so, then went right back and picked up the yelling where they had left off.

Before Baldwin County had its collective case of the candy ass—before it listened to the puerile maunderings of empty-headed deer hunters and closed the fall season—I could have gone down to the turkey racket and done something about it. Or, if I had been two miles north in Clarke County—which has not yet put its brains in a sack and lost the sack—I would have been able to do something about it. Where I was, as it was, all I could do was listen.

They finally finished the argument—you couldn't tell from where I stood who won the debate—and walked off in a body, still exchanging insults back and forth. I waded around and gathered the decoys and then addressed the problem of getting back into the boat.

In knee-deep water it is almost no problem at all. Everything is low enough to allow you to simply step in. Thigh-deep water, coupled with the degree of inherent instability that accompanies light weight, a narrow beam, and a two-inch draft, makes things a little tender for a man in chest-high waders. You are better off getting to the side of a bushy cypress sapling and using the limbs to help you climb over the gunnel.

The boat is almost a marvel. It is a reproduction of the Dan Kidney boats and Green Bay Floaters that first appeared in the marshes at the mouth of the Mississippi River in the late 1890s.

Thomas Staniels of Pilot Town, Louisiana, was one of the early builders who duplicated these boats. The thing I own is called a Staniels Duckboat, is made of fiberglass, and was constructed directly from one of Mr. Staniels's hand-crafted cypress hulls.

I didn't buy it to use. I bought it to reproduce, in wood, and to use as a replacement for a juniper skiff that I had made personally and had hunted out of for almost thirty years.

The replacement was done some years ago, and there is almost no chance now that I will ever reproduce this thing in juniper. The fiberglass model is even lighter than juniper, is stronger, and if there has ever been an example of a maintenance-free item, this boat qualifies. The payment for all its other good qualities is an inherent instability, usual in all pirogues. But on the basis of ease, convenience, and laziness, it is reminiscent of Alexander Pope's classification of the three stages of sin: "First endured, then pitied, then embraced." It is now firmly established as an inhabitant of stage three.

Paddling back across the pond that morning, I fell to thinking how things had gotten to this stage, what inherent streak of blatant and feckless irresponsibility had caused me to backslide, and just exactly when it was that I first came to an old man's crossroads and wandered down the wrong turn.

Because it has been a wrong turn. The old model, while not part of my boyhood, was clearly a part of my young manhood. It spanned nearly the whole of a working career and a substantial part of one of my many avocations. In its building, use, final disposal, and replacement, it involved a remarkably diverse cast of characters.

The wrong turn, like Peter's multiple denials that preceded the biblical cock's crow, is now some several years behind me, and a substantial number of the cast of characters who were involved with that first boat are now residents of that Great Wood Yard in the Sky.

Before all of us get there—and because the tale of that first skiff is partly the tale of an industry, partly that of a career, and partly that of a social system that constituted a minor slice of Americana—it may be worth a look.

Everything in life tends to be relative. At this point, fifty years really doesn't feel as if it were all that long ago. But a point in time fifty years before I got out of school and got in the bush business predates the movement of the lumber industry from the lake states to the South, and that, even to me, seems to have been a very long time ago indeed.

Not that the length of time has any real bearing, because things that concern themselves with people are ageless. I recognize that the relative importance of the Drum and Bugle Corps in the Order of Battle has changed since then, walls being no longer breached with trumpets, but people have been people since Joshua fought at Jericho.

2

The Wood

THE LUMBER INDUSTRY in the United States began in New England—even before the colonies became the United States—and for nearly two hundred years was centered in Maine. In about 1850, it shifted to New York, and by 1860 had moved to Pennsylvania. From about 1870 until the mid-nineties, it was centered in the lake states. For all of this time, the species of preference—and, in fact, the only tree that counted for much of anything—was eastern white pine.

There was a moderate amount of hardwood cut for furniture, although the really high-class furniture was made of mahogany or rosewood. Species like Walnut or Cherry were considered suitable for farmers maybe, or perhaps for the deserving poor, but good furniture, furniture suitable to be sat upon by blue bloods, had to be made of imported woods.

The lifeblood of the construction segment of the sawmill industry was white pine. It had been white pine ever since the English agents first marked mast and spar trees in New England with the King's Arrow. The only trouble with white pine is that it pretty well stays north of 40 degrees of latitude, and most of it is east of the Mississippi River.

There is a western white pine, but you have to go as far west as Idaho to find it. There is also the sugar pine in northern California. Both are wonderful trees, and both have a wood at least as good as that of eastern white pine and, for many uses better.

But both suffered from what, in 1880, were some crippling defects:

They were too big, they grew in terrain that was too rugged to log easily, and they were too far away.

Logging in the 1880s was largely done by muscle—muscle belonging either to man or animal. Trees were cut down with crosscut saws, which, until about 1885, were made with no raker teeth to move the sawdust out of the kerf. Some of the laughably high stumps you see in the old photographs were not left that high through trifling carelessness or to give office-seekers a place from which to deliver political speeches. A high stump had to be left so that the sawyer could get his back into the work in order to pull the saw through the cut, and this was impossible if the stump was cut down at ankle height.

After the trees were cut down, they were bucked into logs, in place, and skidded to the long-distance transportation system by either horses, mules, or oxen. The purpose of skidding is to move the usable parts of a tree from the stump to the long-distance transportation system that takes it the rest of the way to the mill. If your long-distance transportation system was by water, the system was already in place when you began the logging job. If it was by land, then the only viable system at that time was rail. Railroads can only operate on reasonably flat ground, and if they don't already exist, somebody has to build them.

Out in the woods, where the trees are, somebody always had to build them.

It is fifteen hundred miles from Michigan to Idaho. Airline, and airline distances, were academic in the days when there were no airplanes to airline in, so when the white pine in the lake states was exhausted, the industry had exactly two choices.

The first choice was to move some fifteen hundred miles to the mountains, build railroads in unsuitably rough places, and struggle to log and process trees that were too big to be handled by existing logging systems. (Old growth western white pine has diameters of as much as eight feet, and sugar pine is even bigger.) Then, after struggling to log and mill the oversized trees into lumber, they could spend all kinds of freight money to ship the lumber more than fifteen hundred miles to get it back to market.

The second choice was to go someplace closer, flatter, and nearer to the market (someplace that grew trees of a size that could be handled with existing systems); disregard the fact that these trees were not white pine; and tell the sales force to shut up and sell the kind of lumber that the mill could make.

From Michigan to Mississippi is five hundred miles. The land is mostly flat to gently rolling, and logging railroads could be built for $1,000 per mile. Timber volumes were such that a million feet of logs could be moved for every mile of railroad built. Log sizes were comfortable. Best of all, the economy down there was still flat on its ass. Three of the states in the Confederacy had been occupied by federal troops until 1877, and most of them were still suffering from at least a mild case of Reconstruction in 1890.

Millions of acres of virgin longleaf pine could be bought for a stumpage price of a dollar per thousand at volumes of ten thousand feet per acre, and the land under the trees was thrown in for nothing when the timber was purchased.

Because we were then, and still are, a nation of confidence men, lumber company sales forces were able to convince the customers that they had really wanted longleaf more than white pine all along. They just didn't know enough to ask for it.

Mill after mill, company after company jumped on the bandwagon and moved. For the next twenty-five years, from 1895 to 1920, the lumber industry in the United States had a Southern accent.

There is a curious parallel here. The previous twenty-five years, from 1870 to 1895, marked the period of the long-range cattle drives in the American West, which have been the subject of millions of words, hundreds of movies, and have created that genre known as the "western"—considered by many critics to be the only universal, international art form. There are Japanese westerns, Italian westerns, even Indian westerns—turban, not tomahawk.

The logging business has none of the charisma of punching cattle or six-gun justice. There is little chance that there will ever be woodsy epics with logging superintendents being played by John Wayne–types or that suburbanites in Memphis will begin to affect black slouch hats and crosscut saws at cocktail parties, like the cowboy boot craze west of Arkansas. There will never be double-bitted axe standoffs at anybody's corral, and Hollywood will never show two sawhands, eyeball to eyeball, in the dirt street in front of the sawmill commissary inviting one another to draw—in Japanese.

Two industries, coming almost back to back, both of relatively minor impact, neither lasting more than a single generation, with one leaving behind it an international art form and the other vanishing like wind-blown leaves.

A splendid example of the efficacy of ink and public relations on the one hand and a lack of it on the other.

The industry came south for longleaf, set itself up for longleaf, and concentrated on longleaf. Not only did longleaf satisfy all the requirements of size, distance, and terrain, but it had almost no understory, which made logging easy and had the added advantage of exuding resin in salable quantities. This sometimes meant that the sale of turpentine rights could pay for building the railroad.

Longleaf and slash pines both exude oleoresin in commercial quantities when wounded. Oleoresin, called resin, is collected in barrels, carried to a distillery, and heated. Turpentine is driven off in the form of vapor, which is then condensed into a liquid and sold as the turpentine we all know. The residue, now called rosin by everybody but Dizzy Dean, who called it "rawzum," has a wide variety of uses, two of which happen to be helping people to play violins and to throw curveballs.

There are other southern pines that were and still are used—some of them now to a larger degree than longleaf. There were and still are a couple of other conifers used as well, minor species having minor uses. One of these minors is cypress; the other is Atlantic white cedar, known locally as juniper.

In some locations, cypress was major rather than minor and was used all across the region long before the official lumber industry came south. It has the characteristic of being extremely durable in water and for years was made into shingles, shutters, doors, boats, and anything that was going to be used under adversely moist conditions. It had another advantage as well, at least in those specimens that grew along major river systems: It was the easiest tree of all to steal, because you could girdle and kill it one year, then cut it down and float it out during the next year's high water.

Juniper was the premier small boat material from the time the American Indians first made it into dugouts until fiberglass came along after World War II and changed the boat business.

Commercial Timbers of the United States gives juniper a specific gravity of .31, lighter than any other commercial species except northern white cedar. It works well under tools, shrinks only a little, and is fairly easy to bend. It is not nearly as resistant to decay as cypress, although it is comfortably resistant, but it weighs thirty-five percent less, and that thirty-five percent is always with you.

Nowadays, light weight in boats has pretty well been relegated into the interesting-but-not-critical category, except for those people who portage canoes around rapids.

People using a boat to run from place to place simply beef up the horsepower hanging on the transom to overcome any extra weight and press on. Things have even gotten to the point that the ancient occupation of boat paddling by bream fishermen has been replaced by the electric trolling motor, even though the electric trolling motor cannot bait the hook, take off the fish, pass the bottle, and deliver selected examples of rural wisdom. A modern bass boat, fully equipped, has approximately the same amount of electronic equipment as did a World War II submarine. But back in the early days, when travel by water was effected either by wind or muscle, light weight was everything.

Atlantic white cedar is a coastal species. It occurs as far north as Massachusetts, but never much more than seventy-five miles inland and, as far as I know, does not grow west of the Mississippi at all. Along the Gulf Coast there has never been very much of it, and long before the advent of the lumber industry, its particular properties created a demand that appears to have operated almost irrespective of ownership or geography.

A juniper of a size to produce boat lumber had the same characteristics as a bee tree. It belonged to the man who found it. But because it grows along minor streams rather than along big river swamps, after the country got settled and the lumber industry became operational, it did not lend itself to casual theft as readily as cypress.

Occasionally a sawmill would cut a little, mostly for officers of the company or friends of high rank. From time to time a small ground mill would specialize in juniper logs cut on a custom basis, or maybe even cut a week's run of logs specifically for the boat business.

People not in the business have little appreciation of the difficulty involved in asking a sawmill of any size to wrench things around to cut a small, special lot of an unusual species.

The first job I had, fresh out of school, was with an organization called the Alger Sullivan Lumber Company. They had moved down from Michigan, bought a half-billion feet of virgin longleaf in lower Alabama in 1900, set up a mill, and begun operations.

By the time I went to work for them in 1949, they had realized they were growing more timber than they cut. They intended to be in business for the long term, so had begun to concentrate on two special items: export timbers (nine by nine inches and bigger, thirty feet long and longer) and what was, and still is, called bowling alley stock.

In a bowling alley, the part at the foul line where you are apt to loft the ball is maple, and so is the other end of the alley, the part right under the pins. In the middle—and it is a long forty-foot middle—the alley is floored with inch-and-a-quarter-thick pine, cut three inches wide and standing on edge.

Both export timbers and bowling alley stock were high-volume, high-profit items, and every other thing normally cut in the sawmill was fit in around their schedule. The mill cut no hardwood at all, except for rough two-by-six oak to make bridge flooring for the log trucks. This was done all at once, on an odd Saturday here and there, after a day's run of oak logs had been saved up.

Asking the mill to cut a one-boat order of juniper—with the resulting upheaval of normal operations that such a thing would cause—is a request that is unreasonable to the point of outrage, even though the Company lands were cruised with seven million board feet of juniper along one major creek.

Such a request would require that a single truckload of a separate species be logged, transported, run through the mill by itself and, worst of all, handled through the dry kiln in a separate charge. It would have to go through the planer mill separately, be put in the finish shed separately, and stored separately.

All of these things are within the realm of possibility. So is asking an ice cream company that is in the middle of a five-thousand-gallon run of vanilla to stop and make one half-pint of strawberry. The analogy is precise.

As a consequence, unless you are the son of the owner of the sawmill or have concrete evidence of some particularly horrible crime the owner has committed (something of the same magnitude as multiple treason or being caught in bed with an entire boys choir), you either have your juniper cut in a small ground mill somewhere, or you know somebody who knows somebody.

The man I knew was Leon Mosley, but what I didn't know at the time was just how much clout he really had, or that sometime later on, I was to become his son-in-law.

3

The Donors

THE SAWMILL BUSINESS, like the army, tends to create a vocabulary all its own. One of the sayings common to most of the sawmill and logging business is that any man who owes the devil a day's work will be paid off in sons-in-law.

There have to be exceptions to any rule, and Leon Mosley has to be the most notable of the many exceptions, because there is no way this man ever owed the devil a day's work. His collection of sorry sons-in-law—he had two daughters—simply has to be one of those one-in-a-million anomalies.

He had been with the sawmill for twenty-five years when I met him. He was then the assistant lumber salesman working out of the main office. One of his duties was handling the retail sales window.

An old-fashioned southern sawmill was loaded with stiff-necked practices, and one of the more common of those was that there was no such thing as an in-house promotion. The job you took the day you got there was the job you held the day you left, and it was a matter of no consequence to the management if those two days happened to be thirty-five years apart.

Promotion from within, like disrespect to the flag and a hatred of motherhood, was a thing outside the scope of acceptability and was simply not done.

I had very little official contact with Leon Mosley during the early part of my tour with Alger Sullivan. Beginning foresters sel-

dom went into the office; they were allowed in there only in the
event of extremely rainy days (rainfall, say, at about the level of
an inch an hour) or on Saturday mornings, when everybody
worked half a day. Otherwise they were expected to be out in the
woods, where they belonged. The times they were in the office,
they were expected to be working on maps, adding up tally
sheets, or doing growth data calculations, not prowling about
the building having idle conversations.

The sawmill office was run on approximately the same set of
guidelines for discipline you would expect to find in the stan-
dard operating procedure of a row galley in the Byzantine navy,
and if it had not been for the periodic appearances of Mr.
Walker Pruitt, it would have been a grim and gloomy place indeed.

Mr. Walker Pruitt was the Company surveyor, who occasionally dropped by on a Saturday morning to talk over one or the
other of those recurring land line problems that are endemic to
corporate holders of timberland.

Way up at the very top of the corporate list of those criminal
acts expressly forbidden to employees of the Alger Sullivan Lumber Company was smoking in the office. This was long before
the days of having a smoke-free workplace because of medical
reasons. It was done because the president of the company did
not smoke, considered a lighted cigarette to be an object with a
fire on one end and a fool on the other, and therefore had no
sympathy with, or appreciation of, the wishes or desires of the
fool concerned.

Mr. Pruitt would come in, go back to the woodlands area of
the office, spread one of the maps on top of the drafting table,
and get out the field notes of land lines he had run during the
past week.

The office draftsman, those of the timber markers who were
in the office, and anyone who had been called in to go over
whatever discrepancy Mr. Pruitt had discovered, would gather
around the table. Mr. Pruitt would reach in his pocket and bring
out his pocket knife, a box of wooden kitchen matches, and the
biggest and most ostentatious cigar you ever saw in your life. He
would clip the end of the cigar, light a match, warm the cigar
from end to end, put it in his mouth, and strike another match.

He would point at the map with his free hand, talk around

the cigar, point with the hand that held the burning match, and continue the conversation until the match burned down to his fingers and went out. He would then put the burned stub back in the box, reload with a fresh match, strike it, and continue the conversation.

For the next ten minutes you would swear he was at the point of lighting that cigar every instant. The collection of people at surrounding desks would be tortured nearly to the point of frenzy. At the close of the session, he would put the partly used box of matches and the cigar, still unlit, back in his pocket and leave.

The sigh of relief rising from the entire office as he left would have been audible at sixty yards.

He did it one Saturday just as we were leaving to go to lunch and, on the front steps of the office, I asked him if he ever intended to light that cigar. He told me he had been deviling those old maids in the office (most of them were male old maids) since before I was born, and that he had never lit a cigar in there and never intended to. He said I was like most of the young men he knew, careless and irresponsible. He said we should pay more attention to instructions and strive for accuracy—that the rules didn't say you couldn't light matches or warm cigars in the office; they only said you couldn't smoke there.

Leon Mosley was part of a regular group from the office who ate lunch in the hotel dining room most Saturdays. Lunch on Saturday and Sunday were the only two meals I usually ate in the hotel dining room, although I lived in the hotel. The timber markers (both of us) ate a separate, very early breakfast; ate sandwiches in the woods at noon; and got back too late for the regular meal at supper.

Our supper (no one called it dinner then) would be left on the end of the table, served on a plate with a napkin over it to keep the flies out and the warmth in, neither effort being much more than partially successful.

A lot of weekends were devoted to fighting woods fires in the afternoons, and breakfasts, even on weekends, were generally eaten in waves. As a consequence, there was remarkably little opportunity for cultivated, intellectual conversation at meals (unless you talked to yourself), except for Saturday at noon. At these Saturday lunches I was severely outranked by everybody at the table, and fifteen to twenty years younger than almost all of them, so most of the time I simply ate lunch and left. But it was also the most contact I had with Mr. Mosley, and it gave me an opportunity to get to know him a little.

The relationship between future sons-in-law and their prospective fathers-in-law, while not specifically antagonistic, is, at the very least, mildly confrontational. The prospective son-in-law intends to rob the nest of one of its fledglings, and the prospective father-in-law is interested in maintaining the status quo, even though he began his own nest by robbing a fledgling from someone else.

Leon and I became friends later, and to tell the truth, there was very little jostling even at the beginning. This was very largely due to him and to his temperament, because to paraphrase Will Rogers: I never met a man who didn't like him.

Soft spoken, low key, a consummate deadpan joker—so long as the humor was gentle and no trace of ridicule was in any way involved—he was the kind of man who had only to look up to enter a conversation. The person talking at the time had a tendency to stop so he could find out what Leon was going to say.

As a salesman, he was an absolute menace to your pocketbook. Not that there was the least smidgen of high pressure; his specialty was to come from the other direction. Simply by standing there and being helpful, he ended up selling you more lumber than you ever expected to buy when you walked in there.

Alger Sullivan sold what was arguably the best lumber in the world at that time and had never advertised a day in its corporate life. The company conducted business in the same way as does Rolls Royce and the Purdey shotgun people. If you didn't already know about their product, that was your fault, and they felt no obligation to correct your ignorance. If you did know about it, then you already knew it was the best, and it was therefore not necessary to advertise.

In point of fact, the first time they ever drew attention to themselves was in 1950, when they put an inch-and-a-half ad in the *Southern Lumberman* that said, "Alger, Century, Florida" inside a circle about the size of a half-dollar, with no explanation at all. Didn't say whether they sold lumber, butter, or diamonds.

You were supposed to know already, and if you didn't, you were so low class that nobody cared whether you bought any of their lumber or not.

The company had come south in 1900, bought a half-billion feet for a half-million dollars, built the mill, and begun operations. In 1911, they bought an additional 350 million feet for another half-million dollars, stopped operations on the original purchase, expanded a second mill, and moved all logging operations to the new timber.

The new purchase was only sixty miles or so north of the original setting and was on far less land, which in those days was an advantage. The land in those days, having been thrown in with the timber as lagniappe anyway, was scheduled to be disposed of after the timber was cut. The less you had to dispose of, the better off you expected to be.

They cut in the new timber from 1911 to 1923 (when they considered the later purchase to be cut out), moved back to the south end, shut down one of the mills, and took up operations where they had left off in 1911.

They came back to a far different world from the one they had left twelve years earlier.

Between 1911 and 1923, log standards had changed, and a smaller tree was salable. The industry was within a year or two of moving to the West Coast—the old growth pine was virtually gone by 1925—and the industry already had one foot on the road.

Here then was a lumber company with 150,000 acres of untouched virgin timber, long since paid for out of profits (the northern purchase had overcut by almost a hundred million feet), making lumber of a grade and quality that nobody else in the industry could touch with a twenty-foot pole.

When Leon Mosley came to Alger Sullivan in 1924, this was the kind of lumber he was privileged to be asked to sell.

Nobody ever said Alger Sullivan was easy to work for, no employee ever had to have the help of strong backs to transport his salary to the bank at the end of the month, and there was never a complaint that things would have run smoother if the company had not been so subject to attacks of scandalous generosity. They considered the matter of philanthropy to be the business of the Ford Foundation. They were in the business of selling lumber, and the lumber they sold was the best in the world.

I went into Abercrombie and Fitch one time years later, told the clerk I was an Alabama turkey hunter, and that never in my life did I ever expect to have the money to own a Purdey shotgun. I stated that I had not come in there with any intention of posing as a potential Purdey customer, for I was not, but that just one time, I would like to hold one.

He could not have been more generous and courteous, and he appeared to spend as much time with my trifling amount of no business as he would have spent with a man who had come in to buy two matched pairs.

I have seen Leon do exactly the same thing at the retail window in the Alger office with a black-hatted farmer in tattered overalls, who was buying what amounted to half a pickup load of No. 3 lumber to repair his chicken house.

When a man is selling the best there is, regardless of the nature of the product, it tends to give him a relaxed confidence in himself and his material that is impossible to counterfeit. Couple this confidence with the capacity to make every customer think his business is the most important thing you are going to do all week, and you have people driving away loaded down with amounts of lumber or shotguns or shirts that they had absolutely no intention of buying when they came in.

He did the same thing with me in a different fashion when it came to boat lumber. I had become his son-in-law—had been, as a matter of fact, for more than two years—and on one of our visits, I made the remark in idle conversation that one of these days I would like to have a fishing skiff made of juniper.

It was one of those throwaway lines like, "Next reincarnation I am going to come back as a cat," or like the one that begins, "If I were duty officer of the world . . ." Those things said principally for effect and recognized to be wholly without substance at the time you say them.

The next time we visited his house, he informed me that my boat lumber was stacked in the rafters of his garage.

It was. Sixteen-inch-wide juniper boards, fourteen feet long, surfaced on both sides, the boards were five eighths of an inch thick, and there was not a knot in the pile.

Softwood lumber today is sold in grades, and southern pine

lumber has as its top grade something called "C and Better." Not too many years ago, there was a grade called "B and Better," and some years before that there was a grade called "A," but as we have moved more and more into second-growth timber, we have had to combine some of the grades. There are too many of us. We all can't have our lumber cut from 300-year-old trees, even if we all had the money to pay for it.

Juniper is one of those needle-bearing trees that is not properly a hardwood or a softwood, even though the wood qualifies as soft. But the grade of the boat boards stacked on the rafters in the shed had to be A and Better, and I know there ain't no such grade.

Unless you happen to be Leon Mosley's son-in-law.

The logging crew foreman had had somebody pick out a juniper that would yield 16-inch clear boards and cut it down. Somebody kept it separate on the log deck, hauled it in on top of one of the trucks, and picked it out of the log pond as soon as it was dropped in. It had to go through the mill by itself, go through the dry kiln as a separate entity, get through the planer mill and the finish shed undisturbed, and then be delivered to his house by truck, all by itself.

The analogy I used in the previous chapter applies. Right in the middle of a five-thousand-gallon run of vanilla, five separate foremen had been willing to stop the operation to make a half-pint of strawberry on Leon Mosley's unsupported word. And to put the frosting on the cake, not even make it for *him*. Make it for one of his sorry sons-in-law.

And all this trouble was not taken for the man who owned the business. Nor taken because of the degree of power or political clout behind the request. Five separate mill and logging supervisors had conspired to do this favor for Leon Mosley because there were that many people who liked him and because he had asked a favor.

It is the kind of thing that—if it could be reduced to half a sentence—a man ought to have on his tombstone.

I understood all this at the time and I understood something else: that all I could do was thank him. In the situation we were in at the time, there was no way I could take the lumber out of his shed, let alone build a boat out of it.

I had left the sawmill and had taken a new job in a different state. We lived in an apartment, upstairs over the county newspaper office on the courthouse square, a hundred miles north of the sawmill. I could have borrowed a truck and hauled the lumber up there, but I would have had to pile it on the sidewalk in front of the building after it arrived.

But we were a lot farther down the road. I now owned the lumber. It was simply a matter of waiting for the right set of conditions to develop to be able to use it.

Things had progressed to a point considerably past the matter of ownership. The next steps could concern themselves with opportunity and the matter of time and place.

4

Location and Design

ONE OF THE MANY THINGS that ought to be recognized by employees of most major corporations is that by and large, job transfers cannot be refused.

If the transfer is accompanied by a promotion, it is the poorest possible politics to refuse it, for you will then brand yourself as a stay-at-home and may never be offered another move.

If the transfer is a punishment for poor performance, you are being sent to whatever is the corporation's equivalent of Siberia, and you will not be allowed to refuse it (the alternative for refusal being dismissal).

If the transfer is for the convenience of the organization, then you would become a self-serving, selfish son of a bitch and let the side down if you did refuse it.

Consequently, the only viable course of action when you are offered a transfer is to accept the move with alacrity and smile all the way to the new location.

The move I was offered, the one that got us out of the apartment over the newspaper office and off the courthouse square, had nothing in it but good.

It was to a faster league that had a bigger variety of operations and was in a different timber type, selling a different product. I was to boss the job (although one of the people I was to boss was not only forty years my senior but was one of the legends of the business), and the move came with a company house that rented for ten dollars a month.

Next to the house was the office and attached to the office was a shop. The shop was of a size that allowed me to take over one corner of the building and turn it into a boatyard. This gave me, for the first time in my life, the single thing that is absolutely required for any person who intends to work in wood: a place to set things up.

I had nothing but hand tools, and not a lot of them, for that matter, but the absence of a lot of tools is not a serious deficiency.

What is absolutely critical is that there be a vise (to hold things steady while you work on them) and a place to leave things in process when you have to go do something else.

Give a man a bench with a vise, a couple of handsaws, a plane or two, a hammer, a brace and bit, a screwdriver, and a square, and he can build a house full of furniture.

Add electricity, which opens up the world of power tools, and he can get fancy and become a cabinet maker.

Give him twenty thousand dollars' worth of power tools and no place to use them, and he is an equipment collector.

I had a bench, a vise, the barest minimum of hand tools, a vacant corner to work in, a source of electricity to light the work place and to run the quarter-inch drill (the only power tool I possessed), and I borrowed a plane.

The company house and the shop/office was located on company land, two miles from the nearest house and three miles south of the town of Green Bay, Alabama, a hamlet so small it had the town marker at the side of the road on a single sign. The words Green Bay were painted on opposite sides of the same board.

But we were moved, I had both of the necessary requirements and room to operate, the boat lumber was out of the rafters of the garage and on hand, and the South Green Bay boat works was open for business.

There was one final obstacle. Before the boat works could take up its principal business, it was going to be necessary to build a kitchen table so that the single workman and his wife would not be required to eat from trays held on their knees. This piece of preliminary construction had to come first and did, and in the course of building it, the final components of the boat were assembled.

All I had for the boat were the side boards and the bottom. Sixteen-inch juniper, dressed down to five eighths, is great for parts of boats. But for the stem, seats, transom, and ribs (if you are going to use them), you are either going to have to come up with thicknesses of other sizes or glue boards together. Gluing knot-free, sixteen-inch, five eighths-inch juniper into a thickness suitable for either boat seats or transoms is the equivalent of making papier-mâché out of fifty-dollar bills.

But there was a substitute available—the property of the legendary employee who officially worked for me—in the form of a stack of pond cypress boards cut an inch and a half thick, eighteen inches wide, and twenty feet long.

Taxonomists never seem to be able to conquer their innate proclivity to meddle, and they move species and even whole genera back and forth from one family to another. Plants are put into families on the basis of the characteristics of the flowers anyway. This method of classification puts spanish moss and pineapple into the same family, a decision that automatically removes your confidence to begin with.

But as of this writing, the family Taxodiaceae has only two genera, *Sequoia* and *Taxodium,* one with two species and the other with three. *Sequoia,* of course, has redwood and big tree. *Taxodium* has three, baldcypress, pondcypress, and a single species in Mexico, *T. mucronatum,* one specimen of which, near Oaxaca, is estimated to be more than four thousand years old.

Pondcypress and baldcypress have the two words run together in each case to show they are not true cypresses. To make you even more confused than you must already be, the only true cypresses are the cedars. You should be aware that taxonomists do things like this—run the words together rather than change the names—simply to keep us laymen confused.

None of this buys the baby so much as the tip of a shoelace, although it does make work for dendrology professors in forestry schools; but the lumber in the barn in Green Bay, Alabama, in 1955 was pond cypress, two words, improperly used and improperly separated, thereby giving you ample grounds for litigation if you happen to be the legal advisor of the American Botanical Society.

Inch-and-a-half lumber is called "six quarter" in the hard-wood lumber business, and two six-quarter boards eighteen inches wide and five feet long make a dandy table top. It is still a dandy. I have eaten breakfast from it most mornings of my life.

Six-quarter cypress boards eighteen inches wide make a perfect transom for a wooden skiff as well. Make it out of one piece so that you are spared the necessity of gluing anything together (even in these days of universal outboard motors, the use of which has changed the design of the back end of skiffs to a marked degree).

In the era that lasted from the time of the first dugout canoe until World War II, small boat propulsion was effected principally either by wind or muscle.

Along this coast, a rowboat was commonly referred to as a skiff. It was designed to be rowed, although that term was seldom used. The term most generally used was *pulled*. A skiff is pulled—rowing is that occupation conducted during the race between the Oxford and Cambridge boat crews.

I cannot recall exactly when it was I last saw a skiff being pulled, but it has been a long time. We have grown so used to the outboard motor in its almost infinite variety of sizes that we have almost forgotten how it felt to pull a skiff and how much of it went on.

I had a great-uncle by marriage named Elmer Groue. Uncle Elmer was not noted for his intellectual development, but there have been so many members of this family who have had a constant series of opportunities to be modest about their intellect that even though he joined the family by marriage, he fit in beautifully.

Uncle Elmer achieved a smidgen of local fame early in this century by pulling a skiff from Gautier to Ocean Springs, Mississippi, all the way around that big point west of Pointe aux Chenes, carrying three crates of chickens and a sewing machine. He had bought the merchandise in Gautier, and because the L&N Railroad forbade sewing machines and crates of chickens in the day coaches, he took them home himself.

There has always been something in the air around Ocean Springs. The painter, Walter Anderson, regularly pulled a skiff from Ocean Springs to Horn Island, sixteen miles off shore, to spend a month submerging himself in nature; slapping mosquitos and painting.

A lot of working skiffs were equipped with movable centerboards, pinned either up or down in a narrow well in the middle of the boat and equipped with a mast and a scrap of sail all rolled together. You could step the mast through a square hole left in the triangular seat up in the bows, lower the centerboard, drop the pintle of the rudder through its hook, and turn the skiff into a pretty effective catboat. Not fast enough to race around buoys, maybe, but adequate. Good enough to let a man loll in the stern with the tiller under one arm and move along at a rate at least as fast as he could pull the skiff but with the expenditure of substantially less sweat.

The bottom of a Gulf Coast skiff had the normal gentle curve from the bow to a point about three and a half feet from the stern. At that point, the bottom came out of the water. The stern at the transom was six inches or so above the surface of the water and was substantially narrower, top to bottom, than either of the side boards.

I have never heard this construction discussed scientifically. I can only assume that the less bottom surface in the water, the less friction is experienced, and the easier it makes the skiff to pull. When the outboard motor came along, the gap between the transom and the water disappeared. Again, I have never heard this discussed by anyone who appeared to know what he was talking about, but I can only assume it is for the purpose of helping to keep the bow down.

It didn't really make a particle of difference to me then, and it doesn't now. I intended to build the boat to run with an outboard motor, and the fact that all transoms now reached down to the water suited me if it suited everybody else. I had no plans from which to build the boat—felt no need to have any, as a matter of fact—and intended to build the thing by ear, as it were.

I have some friends in the engineering profession who find that last statement to be incomprehensible. They find it impossible to make a plain table, three feet square with straight legs, unless there is a drawing.

Plans and drawings always seem to get in my way and tend to interrupt the free flow of ideas. Admittedly, I have never built a bridge, other than ones for logging trucks, and most of these were composed of three logs cabled together under each track of the wheels. I have no doubt that for complicated constructions and extensive buildings, these plan aficionados are right and that such subtleties are necessary.

The South Green Bay Boat Company, however, and its heirs and assignees for these last forty years have gone free-form.

You fix the size of the boat by the size of the boards on hand. You fix the size of the piece of furniture by the size of the gap in the house that needs filling, and you really don't need to measure much of anything except the height of the seats of chairs and the tops of tables, which, if they are so much as a half inch off, feel awkward when you use them.

Buried somewhere in my psyche is the feeling that if God had expected you to measure anything, he would have made each of your arms a yard long with half-inch wide fingers on each hand and the nail of one thumb scored in eighths and the other in sixteenths.

The juniper side boards were fourteen feet long; there was an old table in the back corner of the shop that was sixty inches wide, sixteen feet long; and I could nail blocks to the top of this table to bend the sides around. The width of the boat was therefore fixed by the room available on top of this table and the length by whatever came out after the side boards were bent.

The flare of the side boards was fixed by the angle cut on the ends of the transom, which was a single six-quarter board. The flare reduced itself gradually as it came to the stem, which was made of a solid block cut from a cypress fence post.

What resulted was an overall length of thirteen feet, four inches and a fifty-two-inch beam. The word "resulted" is specifically chosen. It did not come from a set of plans but from the combination of board length and table width. Things move along immeasurably smoother if you keep them simple.

With the sides bent and flared, with the outside dimensions fixed by the transom (the stem and the two seats and the whole thing held upside down on the table), the rest of the construction was simply a matter of filling in the blanks, as it were, and talking to the visitors who happened to drop by the boatyard during the construction.

Very early in its career, even while it was in the process of being built, the boat began to exhibit the remarkable quality that would last all its working life: its innate ability to attract the strangest people.

I have seen this happen with dogs and have read of it happening with horses, in that a certain breed or specimen causes people to stop you on the street and open discussions as to appearance, characteristics, and probable actions.

The first of these many occurrences happened just about the time it became evident to the casual bystander that what I was building was a boat and not some other piece of furniture, the ultimate purpose of which had not yet been visible. It came from one of the people who worked for me at the new location, the junior member (next to me, the youngest member), a man who had made it clear to me on my first day that not only was he one of those people who drank, he was one of those who had trouble with lids.

We tend to have two kinds of drinkers in rural Alabama. The social kind are the people who have a couple of drinks before dinner, who sometimes have a tendency to sneak bourbon into football games, and who regrettably have a proclivity to overindulge on holidays like New Year's and other special occasions. And then there are the other kind, the nonsocial kind, the people who are known as lid drinkers.

A lot of loggers are lid drinkers. So are a lot of log scalers, truck drivers, and barge hands. A great many timber cruisers and soldiers fall into this category as well.

The hallmark of the species is that once they open the container that holds the whiskey, they are going to drink it all. It makes no difference whether it is a half-pint, a gallon, or a number two washtub. Once they crack the seal and unscrew the top, they throw the lid away, because it has become superfluous. There is going to be no further need for it.

I do not intend to imply that all of these people drink to excess all the time. Frequently there are long dry periods between containers, and many of them recognize their failing and turn down offers of occasional snorts. These refusals come because they are aware that once they start, they are going to press on to the finish, regardless of how long that may happen to take. They are aware of their weakness and are sorry for it—not sorry enough to quit, mind you, but they have sufficient recognition of the failing to take some mildly remedial steps.

And one of the first flies to become entangled in the boat's web was a splendid example of a man who suffered from an advanced case of lid drinking.

5

Construction and Members of the Cast

WHEN YOU ARE ASSIGNED to a new job, there is a remarkable difference in the reception you can expect to get from the group that is already in place in the organization, depending on your position in the pecking order.

If you come to the group as a new boy, or as a new addition, and if, in the opinion of the existing organization, you have not taken a promotion that somebody already on board deserved, your welcome may be a trifle reserved, but it will never be any worse than lukewarm.

You are felt to be too new to be a threat (unless you happen to be one of the boss's nephews) and, presumably, you can be expected to do part of the work. There will be the normal guarded period of reserved acceptance while people make up their minds as to whether you are so stupid that you might actually constitute a handicap. But on the other side—to balance the reservation—there is the usual sympathy of the downtrodden for one another.

Somebody will point out the men's room and the location of the coffee pot, somebody will introduce you around, somebody will offer a cursory explanation of your new duties or, at least, the duties as they were handled by your predecessor. The climate might be described as one of "Let's watch his swordplay a little while before we turn loose the lions."

Unless you come in as the boss.

If you have come there to lead the group, then you must recognize that a completely different set of ground rules will come into operation. The most prominent characteristic of this set of ground rules is that everyone already there feels it necessary to keep his distance.

You may be one of those leaders who feels compelled to have an introductory meeting, conducting it either as "Let's all win one for the Gipper" or "You play ball with me and I'll play ball with you; you don't play ball with me and I'll stick the bat up your ass." Most introductory meetings traditionally tend to follow one or the other of these two general formats. Either way, you cannot bridge that original gap.

Nobody at that first meeting is going to let you get in his head. They are going to stand there with their faces carefully frozen and polite you to death.

Even the professional ass kissers in the group—and these, like the poor, are always with us—are going to stand mute at the beginning. Everybody holds back.

You are too much of an unknown quantity, and no matter what you say or don't say, they have been bitten before. They are going to wait and see what you do and make up their minds on that evidence. You are going to be categorized on the basis of your actions, and nothing you say at first is going to have the slightest effect on the speed of the classification process.

It is for this reason that I have never believed in holding introductory meetings and as a practice have carefully refrained from any discussion of either baseball bats or Gippers.

The morning of the first day after the transfer from the courthouse square, the man I was replacing introduced me. I said I was glad to be there, said I was looking forward to working with all of them, and left everybody to go about their usual business.

The normal employee complement at that time was seven. The Legend was the overall straw boss and was a combination of oldest resident, final authority on all historical matters, repository of all knowledge concerning the land, and Regimental Sergeant Major. It had been made plain, by inference, that I would do well to issue all instructions through him.

It was an unnecessary suggestion.

When a man is forty years your senior in age, has been working on the same tract of timber for fifty-five years, and has been known to say publicly that H. H. Chapman was a nice boy—albeit a trifle green—the fact that you have been officially awarded a rank one step above him on paper does absolutely nothing to oil the path before you. In fact, it creates a situation that can only be handled properly with velvet gloves and silken reins.

I proposed to control this man with all the force and vigor of butterflies alighting upon new violets. Nobody had to warn me of the need to be careful.

Besides him, there were two individuals whose principal responsibilities were roads and equipment; two who did the timber marking, scaling, and sale inspection; and two who were carried as laborers and did most of the heavy lifting. One of these last positions was unfilled at the time, and the incumbent of the other one had not yet shown up. Privately, I considered this to be a rather poor start—the matter of not showing up for work on the first day the new boss came in—but this opinion was inaccurate.

The start was to be even poorer than I had estimated.

The timber markers had gone about their business, the Legend was busying himself with the road crew at the back end of the equipment yard, and I had just walked down the front steps of the building when I noticed a car approaching the office from across the highway.

Passing the office going north and south was a U.S. highway. Thirty yards east of the highway and parallel to it was a branch of the L&N Railroad. Coming west, crossing both to continue into the driveway of the office was a county road, graded but ungraveled and surfaced only with the natural soil.

A car was approaching the office along this road, slowly, sliding back and forth in the ruts—it had rained hard the night before—and just as it got to the right-of-way line of the railroad, the car slid off the road into the left-hand ditch. Once there, the car slowly and gently lay down on its left side, exactly as if it were tired and was going to sleep.

I walked across the road to see if I could help the occupant. Just as I got there, the right-hand door opened, precisely like the hatch of a submarine being raised, and the late arrival climbed out on the hood and slid feet first across the windshield into the ditch. It was not necessary to ask why the accident had happened. You could smell the reason from ten feet away.

I have, myself, in the course of a long and speckled career, occasionally been guilty of some extremely poor first impressions. In many of these instances, realizing what was happening, I have desperately searched for some spectacularly clever line designed to take the sting out of the moment.

None of these searches has ever been all that successful, but then, on the other hand, none of my first impressions have ever been quite so distressful. Considering what he had to work with, I was absorbingly interested in what he was going to say. He did about as well as anybody—and substantially better than I could have done myself, given the same set of conditions.

Without turning a hair and with as much dignity as a drunken man standing next to a wrecked car in a muddy ditch can exhibit, he said, very quietly, "Why don't you just fire me now and get it over with?"

And I answered, "I make it a point never to fire a man on the first day. Let's you and me decide to talk about it later on."

He had brought his wife along, I suppose to drive the car back home, and at this point the top half of the lady appeared in the open hatch. Although it is not common in backwoods Alabama for ladies to be casually introduced after car wrecks, we murmured the proper platitudes (although I did not wade through the ditch to shake hands). Everybody connected with the affair stood around and spoke of inconsequentials while a tractor was brought across the road and the car tipped back onto its wheels and pulled out of the ditch. He and I agreed we should postpone our discussion of the matter for another time and agreed to meet early the next morning.

He couldn't wait that long.

That afternoon, after the troops had come in from the woods and put things away, I mixed my before-dinner drink and walked over to the new shop. The boat boards had been piled near the table, and I was marking off places on the table top where the blocks would be nailed to achieve the curve in the side boards when Stacey drove into the office yard, saw me at the back end of the shop, and walked over to the table.

I mix a heavy drink. Bourbon and water, mixed at the rate of two shots to the glassful, colors the drink a perfectly recognizable brown and leaves little doubt in anyone's mind as to what there is in the glass along with the ice.

There was no way to hide it, there was no way to pretend it was not mine, because the ice was still unmelted and the drink was obviously fresh. It was just as obviously half consumed, and there was nobody there but me. I was going to be put in the position of counseling an employee on the inappropriateness of drinking on the job and the inherent dangers accompanying the use of alcohol while I had a drink in my hand.

Nobody ever said being the boss was going to be easy.

He was clean shaven, sober, contrite, and said he had to come to get things straightened out before he went to bed. Operating on the principle that says if you can't fix it, live with it, we sat on the edge of the table and talked about inappropriate drinking and poor judgment, while the deliverer of the lecture punctuated the discussion by sipping at his bourbon and water from time to time.

There is a rule of thumb in tactics that says if the operation works, the decision must have been correct. This rule must have been operational because we never had to have the conversation again. I saw him drinking afterward, off the job. He formed the habit of dropping by occasionally on the weekend to visit at the site of the boat construction and even, upon occasion, would be partly in his cups at the time of the visit. But he never drank on the job. If at any time he had to miss a day's work, he would be at the back steps at daylight and would conduct the conversation right in my face so that I could satisfy myself that there was nothing on his breath.

We never talked of alcohol again, nor did I ever feel the need to bring it up, except on one occasion, some months later and in another context.

Alabama, then and to this day, works under some strange rules concerning alcohol. A county in the state has the option of voting itself wet or dry, and even a dry county gets a portion of the liquor tax—not as big a percentage as a wet county, but a portion, nevertheless.

Sin, you see, in Alabama, only becomes sin above a certain dollar level.

The county at that time was dry, but there had been a campaign, a petition for a referendum had been circulated, and sufficient names had been gathered to require the county commissioners to call for an election. The afternoon before the election, after work and past the time when everybody had normally gone home, I saw the crew (minus the Legend) still gathered in the back of the shop near the boat table.

Twenty minutes later, the gathering was still in session, and I began to wonder if this was the beginning of a formal request for something or other. Finally, with my curiosity in full bloom, I walked back to the shop and asked if anything was the matter.

Stacey came over to the door and asked to come in the office. When he got inside, he said they were through for the day and everybody was ready to go home, but they couldn't leave because I had not yet told them how I wanted them to vote.

This used to be awfully common in the logging and sawmill business. Not only was it pretty normal, but in rural counties there was a method in place that allowed the boss to tell, after the fact, if his instructions had been carried out.

When they handed you the paper ballot at the polling place, you signed your name on a numbered sheet, officially to show you had properly identified yourself to the poll watchers, but there was a between-the-lines agenda as well.

Down at the bottom of the ballot, on the left-hand side, was a black seal about the size of a quarter. Under that seal, if it were peeled off, was a number that corresponded to the number next to your name on the identification sheet.

You had to know election officials to get it done, but there are always interested election officials in one way or another, and it was always possible to get a look. It was considered only proper that a man needed to be able to find out if he'd gotten his money's worth, or if his instructions had been carried out, whichever case applied.

I did not know all this at the time, and I was still young enough to be shocked and outraged at the idea that people actually told other people how to vote. So I spent some time going over the sanctity of the ballot, the duties of a citizen, the necessity for a man to make up his own mind, and, having done so, the corresponding duty to fearlessly vote his convictions.

Considering the background and prior experience of the group—all unknown to me at the time—they must have felt that not only was I naive, but that I had only one oar in the water as well. But nobody was impolite enough to say either.

After the civics lesson, and when only the two of us were left in the shop, Stacey told me he was glad to hear I felt that way. He said he knew I drank, felt sure I was going to vote wet, and was delighted to find out I didn't expect him to do the same. After all these years I can still quote him verbatim.

He said, "As much trouble as whiskey has caused me in my life, there is no way I could go up there and vote for it. I can't vote for whiskey, and the only way I can vote against it is to vote dry."

I am convinced he voted against it, and it would not have made a particle of difference in either the way he felt or the way he voted if he had been knee-walking drunk at the time he went to the polls.

A man of integrity, whether he suffers from lid trouble or not, has certain lines that he will not cross, and there are no circumstances that will cause him to cross them. Stacey was then, and is now, a man of integrity.

This being so, all rules and conditions apply. One of the conditions is the fact that there is no known instance in which integrity becomes soluble in alcohol.

6

Construction
and Co-Stars

EVERY ONE OF US, at one time or another, finds himself
outranked; and most of us, sooner or later, find ourselves reporting to an individual who appears
to us to be wholly unsuitable because of age, regardless of what qualities the appointing officials may have had in
mind when they selected the person for the position.

One of the more striking examples of such a situation is
found in the case of the fifty-year-old master sergeant, loaded
with experience and decorations, who finds himself reporting to
an unlicked cub of a lieutenant in his mid-twenties, freshly grad-
uated from one of the various commissioning institutions.

Such a relationship can go in any one of several directions.
Carefully handled by both sides, the old-timer can train the
young man from what is, officially, an inferior position. The
older man must be able to smother his resentment, if he harbors
any, and the youngster must be intelligent enough to understand what is happening and allow himself to be led from below.

It can happen, sometimes, without the younger man being
aware of the situation, but in that case it is not nearly as effective. If events take this course and it comes to the attention of
higher headquarters, it becomes an indication of insensitivity
and casts considerable doubt upon the intellectual development
of the younger man.

Done properly, both participants understand that all the experience is on one side and that the other side has only official

status to support it. If the younger man has the wit to realize that it can be done without a threat to his position or a diminution of his manhood, it can be rewarding in both directions.

Such situations are not only possible, they are so usual as to be common, and it always comes as a surprise to me to find out how many people are unaware of their existence.

The whole thing, obviously, can fall apart and degenerate into guerrilla warfare, and if this happens, it is almost an invariable rule that the principal loser from such a breakdown is the junior person. What younger people seldom realize is that the higher authority, who has usually been in a similar situation, almost always realizes it is the younger person who bears most of the guilt and very properly places the blame for the failure where it belongs.

It is a relationship that is, in its way, far more delicate than a marriage. It is easier to manage in the army than in the outside world, because the rigidity of the rank structure in the army precludes the younger man being supplanted by the older. Master Sergeants are seldom, if ever, promoted to Lieutenant.

It was my great good fortune in my dealings with the Legend to be fully aware of the ground rules in such a relationship, having had the good luck to have been trained as a soldier by superbly experienced people of lower rank. The difference this time was that the situation was outside the support of the army's rigidity of rank structure, and the age gap was beyond what would have been possible in any army.

I am exactly the age now that the Legend was when I met him, and to sit here and consider being controlled by a boy of twenty-eight gives me a far better realization of exactly what he did, how difficult it was to do, and what a howling success he made of the whole thing.

The success of the relationship was one hundred percent due to his efforts. My single contribution was to have the wit to shut up and let it happen.

He was thirteen when the century turned and was running a turpentine camp at the age of fifteen and a logging crew at eighteen. In the latter profession, his generation operated under a different set of principles than we are used to today.

To begin with, there was no preceding generation to hand down a set of operational guidelines. Railroad logging of old-growth longleaf began in the twentieth century. Nobody alive had ever done it before, and its practitioners were in the same position in which the fighter pilots of World War I found themselves. It was necessary to teach themselves the rules as they went along, because there were no experienced old-timers to serve as instructors.

Because railroad logging means exactly what it says, it was necessary to have a rail crew as big as the logging crew. The rail crew built rail lines into areas to be cut and took up track in areas that had already been gone over. Today's loggers must build roads, and while there may be some requirement to put the roads to bed afterward, roads need not be taken up and moved to the new location as did railroad tracks. You could leave the cuts and fills, but the rails, the ties, and the bridges had to be picked up and moved. As a consequence, and because so much of the work was done by muscle (belonging to either man or mule), a sawmill that cut twenty million feet a year commonly had two hundred people in the woods, half of them in logging and half in railroading.

With today's equipment, the same volume will be moved with something like thirty people, with technique and capital equipment taking the place of the missing 170 pairs of hands.

The difference then, is that an old-time logging boss did not grow up commanding a few people and a lot of iron. He dealt with and commanded people, and command has a way of becoming habit forming. Command exercised over a long period of time is not only habit forming, it tends to create a mindset that becomes ironlike in its rigidity.

It is extremely difficult to precisely define where management ends and command begins. But a turn-of-the-century sawmill—in which employees lived in a company house in a company town, bought their supplies at a company store, had their water and electricity furnished by the company, traveled to and from work on the company train, and went to the company doctor—was clearly sufficiently controlled to be considered commanded. As a consequence, the style of leadership developed by most of these old-style logging supervisors was definitely one of "I will direct and you will comply."

Start with a man who comes from the generation that had no doubt that it was always right (as was the generation of 1900), a man who is an individual of a self-sufficient nature to begin with. Let him establish the habit of total command of two hundred people in his own fiefdom, the operating ground rules of which he has developed on his own. Let him retain that command under such conditions for nearly a half-century, and then sell the company (including the fiefdom that he has created, controlled, and given his total loyalty) to strangers—and to ignorant strangers at that. Change all the ground rules, reduce the head count he controls to a half-dozen, put him under the supervision of an unlicked whippersnapper forty years his junior, and you have outlined in a few words the fate of a great many logging superintendents all across the South during the last few years of their careers.

I cannot speak for the thought processes of a man who has had this outrage fall upon him, for I have never been that man. I have only been the whippersnapper.

But it was to the Legend's undying credit as a human being and a paragon of resiliency that he handled the situation with grace and wit and good humor and that we became the best of friends despite the handicaps established.

We had some things in common other than the job. He had had one son, an only child, killed in the war at age twenty, and the war had been over long enough for him to outlive any resentment as to why I made it back and his son did not. There may have been a degree of substitution going on, but it was clearly subconscious if it existed at all, because I never heard him mention the boy's name but once.

One afternoon—I can't recall where we were going—he began to reminisce, talked of the boy constantly for almost an hour, shut up in the middle of a sentence, and never mentioned his name to me again until the day he died, a matter of twenty-five years afterward.

We hunted doves together, owned bird dogs together, visited back and forth after I was transferred and he retired, and he died at ninety-three, the only man I ever met who never lost his youthful feeling of immortality.

He would come in the office last thing on Friday, putter around his desk for a minute or two, go to the door, and then turn and say just before he went down the steps, "Tom, unless you need something in the morning, I don't intend to come out here."

And just as invariably and just as carefully I would say that I couldn't think of a thing that looked as if it needed to be tended to.

Those two statements officially closed the week, put the both of us off duty, and left him free to go back in the shop where the boat was under construction and make gently derogatory remarks about the workmanship, every one of which was richly deserved.

Today, I have a small shop. My work is above that of rough carpentry but not up to finished carpentry (let alone cabinet making) but in those days, it ranked just beneath low primitive.

He had loaned me the plane (he transferred ownership of it later) and showed me how to sharpen it and set it up. He was shocked to come into the workroom one evening and find me not only trying to saw a two-inch strip from the side of a fourteen-inch plank with a crosscut handsaw, but not even knowing such a thing as a rip handsaw existed. The Legend was not a finished carpenter either, but on the basis of experience alone, his work was so much better than mine there was little chance of comparison. He was a tremendous help, not particularly in the building itself, but in opening up vistas on things I was not aware were in existence. But while I was willing to accept any comment he might care to make—and did—I drew the line at outside opinions.

He brought a friend to one of our dove shoots one afternoon. The field was just down the road from the office, and after the shoot I invited the both of them by the house for a drink.

Both these old ruins were ex-sawmill foremen, drank what their age group called a toddy, and took a degree of pride in saying they only took one toddy before supper. A toddy was four fingers of bourbon in the bottom of an iced tea glass and a teaspoon full of sugar, stirred in about half a glass of water, with no ice. We had ice in Alabama in 1955, but we had not had it fifty years earlier, when these two started drinking, and sawmill foremen are very seldom on the cutting edge of the avant-garde.

Nor was one drink before supper quite as spartan as it sounded. Four fingers of bourbon in the bottom of an iced tea glass may have been only one drink, but its volume was somewhere between a half pint and a pint, and one was all you needed.

His friend had been the sawmill blacksmith. He still rented the old blacksmith shop at the abandoned mill site and ran his own shop. Earlier that year, he made a pair of log cart wheels for us to exhibit on the front lawn of the office.

Log cart wheels were wooden spoked wheels nearly six feet in diameter with four-inch iron rims and were designed to hold up the front end of logs being skidded by oxen. They were made wholly by hand. The spokes were handmade with a drawknife; the felloes of the wheel cut, curved, and fit by hand; and the whole thing was done to tolerances that allowed the iron rim to be fitted over the felloes only after it had been heated to expansion so it could be driven on. The shrinkage as the iron rim cooled kept the wheel tight and locked the parts together. After the craftsmen who made these things did the individual parts of the wheels, shafts, and axles, and fitted them together, they added insult to injury. They made the rims too.

Taking a man who operated at this level of skill to look at my handiwork as it was in those days was the equivalent of asking Camille Corot over to the house to view your four-year-old daughter's coloring book. But the blacksmith had heard about the boat—at that point I doubt if anybody in the adjacent three townships had not heard about it—and regardless of my level of unease, it would have been rude to object.

The boat was almost at the launching stage. The bottom was done and had been caulked, the seats were in, the final sanding was almost finished, and the thing was out of its blocks and sitting right side up on the construction table ready for painting. It looked like a boat, and if you did not get too close and get too picky about minor gaps at joints—gaps I expected to swell shut in the water—it came reasonably close to being presentable. Not that he would have fallen to the floor in helpless laughter at first sight. He was, after all, drinking my whiskey, standing on my home ground, and had just come from one of my dove shoots. But he could have cleared his throat a little, or inhaled one of those monstrous deep breaths and let it out very, very slowly, so I felt it would be in order to level the playing field just a touch before the fact.

For I did have one card, a single defensive card, a card neither of these two relics knew was in the hand, and because the Legend's expertise encompassed other fields, he was left in total ignorance of the power of the weapon.

In what might properly be called a gentle, preemptive strike, I asked the blacksmith a question. Off-handedly, in the same intonation you use after being asked how many cards you want and you say very quietly, "I'll play these," I said, "Mr. Frank, I understand you used to be in the battalion."

In Covington County, Alabama, there is now and always has been only one battalion. It began as the Covington Light Artillery and was the direct support artillery of the 4th Alabama Infantry back when everybody wore plumes in their hats and wars were fought within the continental limits of the United States.

It is still in operation, now more than a hundred and thirty years since its formation, and service battery of that battalion was then headquartered in the town just south of the office.

I knew the blacksmith had been a member, and I knew he had been in service battery.

The use of the word "the" before the word "battalion" is the key. Among old soldiers, that constitutes the "in" word. That is the special grip and the secret whistle that signifies membership in the order.

Comparative technical skill in carpentry being temporarily put in abeyance, he turned to me and said, "Yes, I was, were you?"

And I answered, "Yes, sir, I still am. I am in headquarters now, but I used to command A Battery."

A direct support battalion of artillery has three lettered batteries—A, B, and C—that are armed with the battalion's cannon, its principal weapon. Rounding out the battalion are two other batteries, headquarters and service, neither of which have anything but small arms and local defense weapons. Headquarters handles personnel, administration, overall command and control, and maintenance. Service battery concerns itself principally with supply and, because artillery ammunition is by nature so bulky and used in such quantities, a very large part of service's duties consist of ammunition resupply.

The logistical support of a battalion in the field—where five hundred people are fed, watered, quartered, and supplied with not only every item necessary for subsistence but every tool required to fight the enemy—is not far short of miraculous.

There has never been an instance since Christ was a corporal in which any supply element of any army in history has received ten percent of the appreciation it deserved for this daily miracle, and they have never gotten two percent of the deserved appreciation from the people who have been the direct recipients of such support.

All line companies of infantry, firing batteries of artillery, and tank companies of armor consider headquarters to be composed of nosy, interfering, overranked busybodies who constantly interrupt the work at hand with silly requests for unnecessary information at wholly inopportune times. They lump all service batteries and support companies in with the household help and insinuate that these soldiers simply stand at the kitchen door, helplessly wringing their hands, while the grown people go off to fight.

This opinion is completely unfair, absolutely unjustified, and almost universally held. It has been held so long that it has become part of the folklore of armies, one of the unkillable myths. Oddly enough, service elements have grown so used to it that while actively disbelieving it themselves, they have come to expect it.

For me to point out to the blacksmith that I was a former member of a Firing Battery (both words capitalized) and to insinuate by a lift of the eyebrows that people in service battery (both words lowercase) simply delivered rations, replaced shoes, and threw aprons over their heads so they couldn't hear the bullets was completely unfair, though not unexpected. He had been living with such insinuations for years and he and I, although two generations apart in years, both knew it.

The fact that this had absolutely nothing to do with building boats was immaterial. What was material was that territorial imperative had been invoked.

I have no idea what he had originally intended to say. I only know what he said.

He made a comment or two about the wood, said it looked as if I were nearly finished, and asked what I thought the boat would weigh. Then the two of them got back in the car and drove off.

Antoine de Saint-Exupery, the French fighter pilot and author, once wrote a marvelous aphorism: "A rose does not know it is helpless. It thinks its thorns are terrible weapons."

Amateur boat builders, when confronted by master craftsmen, have no thorns with which to defend themselves.

But all men are simply little boys who have gotten heavier and more wrinkled. They are no less subject to one-upsmanship at seventy than they were at seven, even if the comment used as the crusher happens to be specious, inaccurate military folklore, and two wars old.

Properly handled, intonations and eyebrows can be infinitely more terrible than thorns.

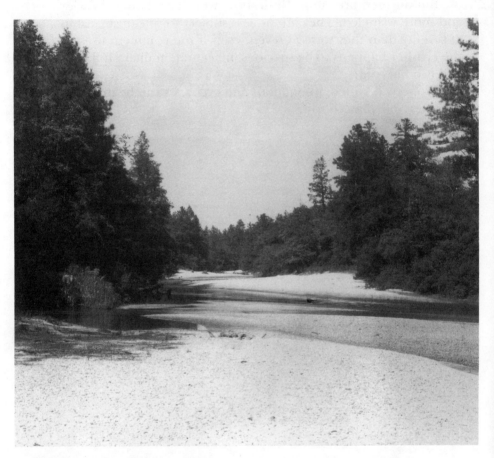

Looking north up Big Escambia
1. The mouth of Spring Creek is found on the left, just in front of a clump of waist-high weeds.
2. The woods road comes in from the left (not in picture). The boat was launched across the gravel bar in the foreground.
3. Bartram's Crossing is located in the middle of the background, where remnants of old piling are apparent in the creek.
4. Most of the trees are juniper.

7

Move and Launch

ONE OF THE WAYS to make sure that anything you build turns out well is to have the luxury of not having to hurry to finish it. Hurrying things to completion is one of the prime causes of sloppy results—almost a guarantee of them—even with something you knew how to do in the first place. If you are feeling your way along with a project, learning as you go, the last thing you need is to be pressed for time to get things finished.

I did not have to carry the specific cross of hurry with the boat. Just before completion and just before seeing if the thing would really float—and even more important, float with people in it—we got notice of another transfer.

So the only hurry involved in all of the construction was the matter of covering the bottom of the boat with fiberglass and epoxy.

Fiberglass is sold in rolls or sheets with the epoxy required to stick it to whatever material it is to cover. Sufficient hardener is included to add to the epoxy to cause it to set up after it is applied.

My wife helped with this; it almost requires two to do it, and you would be better advised to have three, because as the epoxy begins to set, things tend to get a little frantic.

I have always thought that there was never any reason to raise your voice to the ladies. I leave out girl children. Sometimes girl children only respond to piercing shrieks, but grown

49

ladies are another matter. Covering the bottom of a boat with fiberglass sometimes requires you to deliver a great many instructions, some of them conflicting, in a very rapid manner. A dispassionate bystander might conceivably conclude that some of your repeated comments to your helper might qualify as yelling, even when they do not. It is a comfort, therefore, to epoxy a boat in a shop that is two miles from the nearest house, through the woods, so that no misunderstandings can possibly arise through the neighbors overhearing some of the comments.

Not only did the bottom of the boat get covered, but the marriage survived. Two days later, after the covering dried, I painted the boat a dead-grass green with duckboat paint. Construction was complete.

The two decades from 1955 to 1975 were marked by the movement of thousands of acres of timberland in the South out of the hands of old-line sawmills and into the hands of paper companies. There were private tracts changing hands all along, of course, but the major switch in ownership that occurred during this period consisted of transfers from sawmill to paper mill. The company I worked for during this time came to the end of 1975 with a half-million acres of fee ownership, nearly 400,000 of which had come in the first of the two decades, and three quarters of that from sawmills.

The total acreage held by corporations changed very little. What did change was the identity of the corporation.

Among those companies whose lands changed ownership was the concern I had worked for eight years previously, the organization that had owned the juniper lumber that made up most of the boat. They sold out to a consortium of five companies, one of whom was my present employer.

My immediate assignment after the move, and the reason for the transfer, was the requirement to make a rapid examination of the total land ownership of the sawmill—nearly a quarter of a million acres—that was to be divided among five owners. Time was not only of the essence, it was the overriding consideration. The opinion as to the relative values of each of the five parts of the division had to be completed before the split could be effected, and there was a school of thought, held by at least two of the new owners, that the division was already at least a week behind schedule.

As part of the movement of our household effects to the new location, the completed boat was loaded on the moving van with the rest of the furniture, and the boat ended up back under the roof of the same shed it had occupied when it had simply been a collection of unassembled parts.

All of which gave us time to come up with two additional items that would be added to its list of characteristics. First, we had an opportunity to weigh it. Painted and completed, it weighed 104 pounds, seven more than Charles Atlas's notorious 97-pound weakling. And second, as soon as I got through looking at a quarter of a million acres, the move afforded the opportunity to launch the boat on the same stream that grew the tree that made the boards—Big Escambia Creek.

Big Escambia Creek begins in Monroe County—in the southern half of Section 28, Township 6 North, Range 7 East—as Pine Root Branch. It runs into the Escambia River, roughly forty miles southeast of there, two miles across the Florida line. Except for the mile or so when it is still Pine Root Branch, and for a couple of short stretches after that, it runs on lands that belonged to the lumber company, all the way to Florida, and there is not a cleared field on either bank for the entire distance. As a consequence, during periods of flood, it simply gets high—never muddy.

It runs south through all of Township 6 as a normal, lower-coastal plain creek. It boasts a quarter of a mile of swamp on both sides, foot-and-a-half–high banks, and a mixture of sweet bay, black gum, and slash pine timber. All the way down through Townships 6, 5, and 4, it shows signs of old logging ditches dug along tributary creeks where the earliest cutting had been done in the 1880s and the logs floated down to Pensacola. It accepts Corley Creek from the east in Section 9 of 4/7, the junction occurring in an area that held twenty thousand feet of slash pine per acre and more cottonmouth moccasins than anywhere else on the planet.

Two of us marked the timber in there in the summer of 1950, and you had to make up your mind either to kill snakes or paint trees. We painted, but at a speed substantially slower than normal because of the fact that we looked down more than we looked up.

Cottonmouth moccasins—three feet long with a body diameter the thickness of your forearm—have that effect on timber-marking operations. They speed up the metabolism of the markers in a manner inversely proportional to the degree with which they slow down the work, and they play hell with the nervous system at the same time.

Sampey Creek comes in from the east in Section 35, three miles south of the snake pit, and from there to the Florida line—a matter of some twenty miles—the creek becomes not only a different blanket, it is on a different horse altogether.

The addition of Corley Creek doubles the size of Big Escambia, and the waters of Sampey Creek double it again. It becomes a large creek after the additions, with three-foot banks, forty to fifty feet of width, pronounced sandbars and outcroppings of gravel, and a marked change in timber type.

The timber becomes much heavier to oak and has a sprinkling of red bay mixed in with the sweet. This point marks the beginning of the juniper. In some places there are almost solid stands of juniper, five or six acres in size. Because the width of the creek lets in so much more light, in many places the timber directly adjacent to both banks is almost pure juniper.

William Bartram crossed near here in 1775 and describes the crossing as follows:

> In the evening we forded the river Schambe about fifty yards over, the stream active but very shallow, which carries its waters into the bay at Pensacola. Came to camp, on the banks of beautiful creek, by a charming grove of *Illisium floridanum*; from this we travelled over a level country about fifty miles, very gently but perceptibly descending South-Eastward before us . . .

Bartram was traveling along the height of land between the Alabama and the Escambia-Conecuh River basins that would carry the Old Federal Road in the next twenty years. This road crosses Big Escambia just south of the point where it receives the flow of Corley Creek.

The description given by Bartram does not in any way describe the aspect of the land where the Old Federal Road now crosses Escambia Creek. The description given and the ground there are as different as day and night, the ground being typical, lower coastal plain sweet bay and black gum.

The Taitt map of 1772 shows alternate paths in this section, one on each side of Big Escambia, and Bernard Romans, in 1776, gives a width of "about 60 feet" at a still lower crossing.

There are old pilings still in the bed of Big Escambia just north of the mouth of Spring Creek, delineating an ancient crossing; Romans's description of the crossing fits the land there. Spring Creek itself, including the Florida anise trees along its banks, fits the description of Bartram's campsite.

Bartram is notoriously poor when it comes to distances, almost as bad as he is with dates and directions. He was traveling southwest, not southeast, at this point, and his yards are very likely meant to be feet. Big Escambia is not fifty yards wide at any point between its inception and its confluence with the Escambia River.

The body of evidence is therefore quite strong, almost to the point of being conclusive, that Bartram crossed Big Escambia at about the mouth of Spring Creek, spent the night there, and pressed on across the savannahs west of the creek the next morning.

The appearance of the land in there today is the same as that in the picture on page 48 and matches both Bartram's and Romans's descriptions as to creek and terrain.

It was across this gravel bar, there at the mouth of Spring Creek, very likely in sight of Bartram's old campsite, that the boat was finally launched on its maiden voyage, two months after my report on the division of the quarter million acres was made final and accepted and 183 years after William Bartram had passed through on his way to Mobile.

An initial launching at this point had several advantages. Never mind my reckless disregard for the opinions of an ex-sawmill blacksmith who began life as a horse holder in Service Battery—I had substantially more unease about the boat's stability than I had been willing to admit to him, and I wanted the launching to be conducted in private. Besides that, I wanted it in water shallow enough to walk out of if something did go amiss.

Difficulties that arise concerning either boats or aircraft have one principal characteristic in common: Everyone is infinitely more comfortable if these defects first make themselves known while the vehicle is at rest.

A launch on the gravel bar at the mouth of Spring Creek would be in knee-deep water. A woods road ran to within fifteen yards of where the launch would occur, which meant the boat need only be dragged fifteen yards to start. There was a bridge across the creek two miles below the launch point and another one two miles below that. If we had to candy-ass out at the beginning, no one would be the wiser. We could simply drag the thing back to the truck, load it up, and drive home.

I took the position that if we could go two miles, we could go four, so we left one vehicle at the bridge four miles downstream, said to hell with a two-mile safety valve in the middle, went back to the mouth of Spring Creek, loaded up, and launched.

We had two fly rods, a paddle apiece, an axe and a Sandvik bow saw (in case there was a tree across the creek that needed cutting), six cans of beer, and the afternoon.

The boat floated—it floated with a crew of two—it didn't leak a drop, and we found out some things we hadn't known before.

Big Escambia, at the stage of the water then prevailing, has about a four-knot current. A boat going with the current is therefore effectively in dead water all the time and is more difficult to handle than when it has movement through the water. While four knots is not all that much current, it is somewhat too fast to fish in, and you tend to go by the interesting holes too quickly. Most of my fishing had been in oxbow lakes off the river in no current at all, and this matter of motion took a little getting used to.

In order to fish holes properly, we had to ground the boat and wade, which was no real trouble, but it pointed out the fact that you could ride the creek and look at the scenery, or you could fish. It was nearly impossible to do both at once.

Here in the Southeast, we have about as much running water as anywhere in the country, it being most unusual to have a whole section of land without one or more running streams. Such streams in the lower coastal plain are generally narrow, with muddy banks and a mixture of black gum and sweet bay as the dominant species, with a sprinkling of yellow poplar in the drier portions. Big Escambia and some few of the others on the Gulf Coast are the exceptions: shallow, relatively wide, with a brisk current; and in some cases, enough juniper along the bank to give the creek the appearance of being several hundred miles north of where it really is, with hemlock and other northern species along the edges.

We could have run the four miles in an hour and a half if we had not stopped to fish. We found no tree across the channel that needed cutting, and only in a place or two was it necessary to get out of the boat in extremely shallow reaches and push it into deeper water.

And if I had not run us into the hornets.

It was in a fairly long hole of water with not nearly as much current, and Bill had cast to the left descending bank and hung the fly. I was paddling at the time, and because he had cast far enough ahead, there was time to take the couple of strokes and get the boat over to the snagged lure and stick the bow of the boat, and its casting occupant, under as noble a nest of white-faced hornets as you will ever find.

These things build a nest of almost pure papier-mâché, made of cellulose and hornet spit, gray in color, the shape of a football, with some of the better examples (like this one) being about twice the size of a football. The hole the hornets use for entrance and exit is at the bottom of the nest and is about the size of a quarter.

I very nearly put his head right under the hole.

The square name of the American hornet, a member of the wasp family, is *Vesper maculata*, and the book says its sting "causes severe pain," which is the same thing as saying that to be stabbed with a red-hot ice pick can be classed as moderately uncomfortable. It can, but there are whole pages full of other words that describe the feeling far better.

The use of the word "severe," in this context, constitutes understatement to the point of surpassing Mark Twain's comment about the unsuitability of the same word being used in the description of lightning and the lightning bug.

When hornets come out of the nest, they are mad. They wreak their vengeance upon the nearest warm body, animate or inanimate—I have seen them sting a Caterpillar D-8 tractor, and

I am willing to swear that the tractor flinched—and they have no concept of guilt or innocence. They take whatever is at hand.

Bill was in the front of the boat and was handy. The criminal in the stern with the paddle, the careless clod who caused the whole thing, was left untouched.

In addition to the excruciating pain, there is a venom that accompanies the sting that seems to inhibit the clotting of blood. Two or three of the stings on his arms swelled badly, the fingers of his right hand puffed up until they resembled sausages, and the two stings on the lobe of his right ear dripped blood continuously for the next thirty minutes.

Even to those individuals who are not particularly susceptible to bee stings—and there are some horrible stories—ten or twelve of these bites would be very serious indeed.

We chewed enough pipe tobacco to stick on the stings, which may or may not help—but there are enough old wives' tales to that effect that it acts as a placebo, if nothing else. And for the rest of the way down, I worked the paddle as fast as I could while Bill sat in the boat and suffered. Several times he brought up the comment in *Huckleberry Finn* that in the Missouri of the 1840s there was a superstition to the effect that bees wouldn't sting idiots. Bill tended to take the affirmative position in the discussion.

At some time in the afternoon we may have passed the stump that grew the tree that gave the boards that built the boat. There was no assurance that we did, because no one but the logging crew boss who brought it in knew exactly where they cut the tree. But it had to have come from the same creek—and with the exercising of a little imagination, you could convince yourself that you had, in effect, brought the boat back to the equivalent of the Sunny Hill puppy farm.

Such a passage, if it occurred at all, passed without ceremony. I hadn't thought of it before the incident of the hornets, and I damned sure wasn't going to bring it up after the stinging. Nothing that in any way hindered the rapid application of the paddle would have been considered suitable at that point.

It was the Vikings, I think, back fourteen or fifteen hundred years ago, who felt that in order to have a boat properly launched and the sea gods propitiated, the ways should be greased with the blood of enemies.

This boat had no ways to be launched from, being carried to the water across a gravel bar, and our society has grown so formalized and rule-ridden that it has become virtually impossible to make such use of your enemies.

There was, however, blood at the launching. The boat did begin its career by having had dripped upon it blood from the veins of friends.

The Japanese have a ceremony that accompanies the maiden voyages of vessels. There is a wooden cask of sake. The two or three highest ranking people at the ceremony, wearing ceremonial short kimonos and exotic headbands, use wooden mallets to break into this keg (the head of which has been nearly sawed through beforehand) and the wine is dipped from the keg with a special bamboo dipper and poured into little wooden boxes. All persons present drink a toast to the new vessel from these boxes.

Or at least they drink some of it. If you don't drink from the corner of the box, carefully, you pour a lot of the sake down your shirt front and, if you are one of the people in the kimono and the headband, you bathe the front of some of the ceremonial garments as well as your chin. Square wooden boxes make inferior glassware and tend to dribble horribly.

Neither of us was aware of these ceremonial formalities at the time. In our ignorance, we simply carried the boat across the bar, put it in the water, and drank the beer directly from the can on the way downstream.

Sake, drunk warm from the keg, tastes remarkably like the moonshine whiskey made all over rural Alabama. We could have gotten some of that, but without the short kimonos and the headbands, it would probably have been unsuitable.

In any event, except for the matter of the hornets, I can only assume that the sea gods made allowance for our ignorance, gave us constructive credit for both the beer and the blood, and considered the launch reasonably successful.

8

Engine Room

THERE IS A SAYING in artillery battalions that in order for a battalion to operate efficiently, at least two or three of its members must be artillerymen.

The allusion is to the technical aspect of artillery (actually, what the technical aspect consisted of thirty years ago), and the reference specifically addresses itself to the matter of gunnery.

The maxim is one of those things that sounds silly on its face. Presumably, you would think that every person in an artillery battalion would be an artilleryman, but the inference goes much deeper than that. It is used in the sense that is meant when you hear someone referred to as a soldier's soldier or a lawyer's lawyer. It connotates superb professionalism, background, performance, and—in the case of artillery gunnery—what amounts to nearly a mystical ability to know what is going on in places where the individual is not even physically present at the time those events are in process.

A direct-support artillery battalion is supposed to be able to move, shoot, and communicate, and the battalion commander is the person who principally concerns himself with the function of moving.

The commander of a direct-support artillery battalion is presumed to be the best judge of where the battalion should locate itself in order to deliver its fires. He therefore moves the battalion whenever he thinks it is necessary. He alone, of all ranks in the army below that of general officer, is allowed to move upon his own authority. It is not necessary for him to ask permission. He notifies higher, lower, and adjoining headquarters when he is in the process of or has completed the move, but this is done simply as a courtesy and almost always takes the form of a simple, declarative sentence that begins with "I have moved" or "I am moving" to such and such a location.

There is always one single, preeminent, and overriding stipulation, and that is that he must never, ever get his battalion into a position from which it cannot deliver fire on call. It is his only absolute given.

With three firing batteries under his control, he may leave two in place and move one, he may leave one in place and move two; but he may never, never, never have everybody on the move at the same time and consequently be unable to shoot.

If his weapons will shoot fifteen thousand yards, it is preferable to have all batteries emplaced at about midrange from possible targets. This leaves him close enough to shoot deep into the enemy's territory but with ample room to fall back if required. It is impossible to perform in this fashion all the time, however, unless the situation is so static that no moves are required.

As you would suspect, the stipulation "Never get yourself into a position from which you cannot shoot" creates almost an unlimited range of possibilities. The commander has an officer whose principal duty consists of surveying in the positions of the battalion and constantly seeking out alternative position areas. He has officers attached to the infantry who can see the other end of the trajectory and adjust the fall of shot. He has officers in the firing batteries concerning themselves with the weapons delivering the fire, and he has liaison officers with the maneuver battalions who plan fires and notify him of proposed attacks and retreats of the infantry. All of those scenarios are likely to require a move. These officers produce a constant flow of information to assist him in his decisions as to when a move might become necessary and how—and with how many firing batteries—to make it.

In effect, then, such a commander finds it necessary to play "what if" all the time.

Because the guiding precept of American artillery is that if it is worth shooting, it is worth shooting the battalion, the gunnery officer is the man who directs the fires of all three batteries and is responsible for massing these fires at the receiving end.

It is, of course, possible to mass fires by having the pieces that deliver the fire located axle to axle.

Old sailing ships did things that way. Broadsides were delivered by cannon stationed cheek by jowl along the deck, and, until the middle of the twentieth century, naval gunfire in general had the delivering pieces next to one another in turrets.

Field artillery since the Franco-Prussian War in 1870, has overwhelmingly concerned itself with indirect fire, which means the gunners cannot see the target. Especially since the advent of tactical aircraft, the cannon that are firing from within the battery position are required to be dispersed. Consequently, nothing can be massed but the projectiles, and this must necessarily be done at the point of impact.

The officer directing fire, the fire direction officer in such a situation sees neither end of the trajectory. He is often half a mile from the firing batteries on the sending end and five or six miles behind the rounds arriving in the impact area on the other.

If there is only one artilleryman in the battalion, it must be this man.

The battalion commander can be a moving specialist, an administrator, and a keen judge of competency in subordinates. He can possess the ability to inspire confidence in others and make out with relatively minor technical artillery ability.

The individual battery commanders can operate with the same qualities, held perhaps to a somewhat lesser degree.

Forward observers, liaison people, and support people of all description can be specialists in their particular discipline, and things can run reasonably well.

But in the man who runs fire direction, there is an absolute requirement for technical competence in gunnery—nothing else can be substituted. Those fire direction officers who are extremely competent not only do all this, they play in a higher league altogether.

Willie Keeler, the old Oriole infielder, made the comment, "Hit 'em where they ain't."

That comment is not applicable in this instance. There is no place where these guys ain't.

A battalion fire direction center is usually composed of two chart operators, three people called "computers" in contact with the firing batteries, two radio operators, the operations sergeant, and the fire direction officer. Handled poorly, such a group could degenerate into an imitation of Hollywood's version of the floor of the New York Stock Exchange on crash day in 1929—with everybody speaking Italian.

Good fire direction centers are as quiet as mortuaries. Instructions, commands, requests, and the transmission of information is done quickly and is couched in understatement. The tone of the entire operation reminds you of the clipped dialogue heard in those overcivilized drawing room scenes depicted in Noel Coward comedies and produced on the London stage.

In the center of this calm sits the fire direction officer. He is neither at the guns on one end of the trajectory, nor with those people observing the fall of shot at the other, but by some magic of witchcraft—as if he were an entire covey of disembodied spirits—he is somehow able to keep up with all that is happening at either end (or in the middle for that matter) and quite often possesses the wholly unbelievable capacity to detect things that are about to go wrong before they happen. It is very like those persons who are capable of playing chess with a half-dozen opponents simultaneously. You cannot believe a single head can keep that many balls in the air, but it does.

Tal Golson was exactly that kind of a gunnery officer. He had the ability to visualize the entire gun, target, and connection area of the equation at the same time; may have been the perfect, intellectual gunnery officer; and ran one of the worst fire direction centers I ever saw—for the simple reason that he absolutely refused to delegate.

Delegation is infinitely harder for the extremely competent than for those less so. For the true genius, delegation comes very close to being impossible. It is always difficult to stand back and let someone do something that you are able to do far better, especially if you have the official right to step in and do it yourself. But it is necessary in extremely complicated functions in which the sheer mass of detail makes a sole proprietorship a literal impossibility.

There are exceptions, of course. Isaac Stern does not need another set of hands to help him play the violin, nor did Ted Williams need a helper at the bat. These are single-person skills. But no man, not even one as talented in his specialty as Tal Golson, can have the strength of ten, no matter how pure his heart happens to be—and the Golson heart was very pure indeed.

He won the Silver Star with the 3rd Division in France during World War II by calling down artillery on his own position after it had been overrun and from—like the boy on the burning deck—"whence all but he had fled." It was this very belief in his own immortality, this personal conviction that everything was possible, that led him to believe he could be a one-man fire direction center.

He never quit trying. He believed in his very soul that he could really pull it off and, as a consequence, the uproar that came from a fire direction center under his control was audible at fifty yards. A four-hour shift in there left a man as wrung out—mentally as well as physically—as if he had spent four hours in a cage of hungry lions.

They got the rounds out, after a fashion, and during those periods when only one thing at a time was going on it was superb, because he could handle it all, and did. But let there be multiple missions, let there be what are called times on target, let different batteries be firing on targets of opportunity in different directions, and his operation would become the specific definition of bedlam.

He ran his business in private life the same way. He owned the Lone Star service station in Evergreen, Alabama, and when three cars arrived at the pumps at the same time, you could hear the shouting all the way across the railroad tracks on the other side of the depot.

I had met Tal before I was aware of his genius in gunnery, before I ever got in the battalion. I knew him as the manager of the Lone Star service station because it was right across the road from the L&N depot where we used to pick up the Camp 14 payroll.

A great many towns in the rural South were centered around either the train station or the courthouse. Evergreen was centered around both. In the days before the paved road, and in the case of a town not located on the river, the railroad was the only public transportation and almost the only way in and out. Freight, traffic, and passengers all moved through the depot. If the town had been in existence before the railroad came, no stone was left unturned, no promise left unmade, in an effort to seduce the railroad officials into running the track right through the center of town.

The hotel was there to handle the drummers, and most of the downtown businesses were scattered up and down both sides of the track. In Evergreen, not only was all this in place, but U.S. Highway 31 paralleled the track right through the middle of town as well, and the railroad depot was the commercial center of the county.

The lumber company, where I was employed to mark timber and enjoy the distinction of being the lowest man on the sawmill's totem pole, still had one logging camp near Evergreen called Camp 14. A few of the older cutters lived there. The camp still ran a kitchen, and some of the hands lived nearby and caught the morning work bus to the woods from Camp 14.

Friday was payday. The mill paid in cash, and the payroll was made up in the main office at Century, put on the L&N's mail car there, and got to the Evergreen depot along about the middle of the afternoon. The entire timber-marking force—both of us—the company surveyor, and the woods rider who lived near Cook's Store constituted the payroll escort. Two vehicles, four people, with both vehicles armed with one of those Colt .45 Cal ACP revolvers (an item of issue to the army in World War I and used by the post office for years afterward that fired ACP ammunition held in two half-moon clips).

We traveled the eight miles from the depot to the log camp by various routes, on unpaved roads, to fake the payroll bandits off. We successfully outsmarted the villains week after week, and I am still able to take great pride in the fact that there was never an instance of a payroll robbery while I helped guard the funds.

The minimum wage in 1950 was forty-five cents an hour; there were twelve or fourteen people in the logging crew, counting the camp cook, all at minimum wage; and the crew foreman made $50 a week. There is no way there could have been as much as $350 in the whole payroll—it was probably nearer to $300. We could have stuck it under the seat of the jeep when we left Century in the morning and dropped it off at Camp 14 on our way home that afternoon. But that, of course, would have been entirely too dull and prosaic.

Instead, we used to park beside the L&N depot and wait there—armed, dangerous, poised for instant defense, daring any highwayman to approach our escort—and watch the uproar at the Lone Star station while we waited for the trainload of money.

After the Korean campaign, when I had served with Tal for a couple of years and had come to know him as a friend (rather than as a classic artilleryman with one major flaw), I used to go by the station occasionally and visit. We began to hunt together a little. He was aware of the boat construction and launching and was interested. With his temperament, anything that had been conceived and carried out alone was bound to be found interesting, and he brought up the possibility of being the man to furnish the propulsion system.

The matter of leaving the boat in the swamp—strategically located at various points near bodies of water that were to be fished or crossed—or even left in ponds so that it could serve as the container for guns and gear and be dragged along behind you as you waded was intended to be only one of its proposed uses. Even leaving out the matter of taking it down to the bay to hunt ducks, which exposed you to a degree of wind and water conditions somewhat beyond that of calm water, there were the conditions prevalent in upriver traffic.

Moving across and along the river among the tugs and barges, scattering a drove of turkeys and then having the requirement to go home afterward and come back the next morning in the dark, going to gobbling turkeys before they gobbled at daylight, changing your mind at daylight and deciding to go in one direction or another to take advantage of a change in weather conditions—all these situations require a degree of speed in travel that can only be achieved by outboard motors.

It is even more important now. In the early days of the boat's life, Baldwin County had not achieved its remarkable scientific breakthrough. We had not yet realized that we exist here in a completely different solar system: that our water has three atoms of hydrogen to the molecule—rather than two, like Clarke County—that none of the normal laws of physiology apply, and that turkeys would be driven to extinction within six months unless our fall season was closed. Now that we know all this and have evaded the curse of extirpation by closing the fall season, it is sometimes necessary to travel an extra three miles or so to get up to Clarke County, where they don't have the advantage of all this scientific data, and help them shovel their turkeys over the precipice into oblivion.

But it was also important that day at the Lone Star service station, and what Tal was proposing to do was to furnish the motor.

Lone Star was a station in what was then called the Pure Oil System. I have no idea why the Pure Oil people elected to go in the outboard motor business, but they did. They sold a brand called Corsair through their oil dealerships and offered it for sale in service stations all over this area.

Tal had one of these in inventory at the Lone Star station, and he sold it to me after some lengthy negotiations in one of the most unusual transactions I have ever been connected with.

To begin with, we were poles apart in price, but not in the normal sense of a buyer-seller relationship.

He wanted to *give* me the motor, which I was sure he could not afford to do—after all, the Pure Oil Company had not *given* it to him—and my position was that I ought to pay full retail price.

Ordinarily, I haggle very poorly. I cannot escape the feeling that it is rude, somehow, and a trifle insulting, to offer a man less than his opening price. If he did not think the article was worth the quoted price, then he would not have made it. I conduct my own sales on such a basis, and I am always uneasy in making counteroffers to another man. It seems to me to insinuate that I think he is some kind of confidence man who has taken it upon himself to cheat me, and when I make a lower offer, it is to suggest that I have found him out. I understand that this is a minority opinion, that most of my friends and acquaintances think it is a form of insanity, and that all of them are convinced that everything I buy comes at retail plus ten.

Normally, they are right, but in this instance, being on the proper side of the equation, I conducted my business with all the guile and tenacity of a Persian rug salesman whose mother was the eldest daughter of Ebenezer Scrooge. I even sank to the level of asking Pure Oil dealers—people not even members of the battalion—what their retail price was, and then cold-blood-edly using that number in an attempt to drive his selling price even higher.

It is with the greatest degree of satisfaction that I am able to report that I drove his price from nothing up to $160 in proba-bly some of the shrewdest trading since Thomas Jefferson made the Louisiana Purchase from Napoleon.

You should not consider this statement to be bragging. When a man is superlatively gifted, a transparent, spurious mod-esty has a tendency to become cloying and offensive and actually turns into poor taste.

But we traded at the last, and the boat now built, tested, and powered was ready to be launched on its career.

The completion was the result of the efforts and generosity of donors of materials, location for construction, tools, advice and help in building, the necessary muscle for early trials, and a marked degree of financial help in buying the propulsion sys-tem.

With the exception of those ancient dugout canoes, whittled and burned from cypress logs by naked savages, it is unlikely that so insignificant a craft has been able to keep so many people oc-cupied with its construction for so long.

To paraphrase a great Englishman: "Never, perhaps, in the history of boats, have so many, worked so hard, to create so little."

9

Remittance Man

NOW THAT ALL CONSTRUCTION was completed—with the solid assurance that the boat would really float, the capacity to dodge tugs and barges in the dark if required, and the built-in speed to change directions in the middle of a hunt when necessary all in hand—we came to a hiatus.

I was moved again, this time to a location that had no continuing access to the river swamp, thereby removing the set of conditions that called for the flexibility the boat had been designed for in the first place.

We were moved one county north, to a place that had a fall season and that put me close enough to the woods to be able to hunt every day in the spring. But the area I was authorized to hunt did not require the use of the boat to take advantage of the ground.

In American business circles, this is called an excess of capacity in a weak market. In today's climate, it would call for what has come to be known as downsizing.

Downsizing a one-boat fleet tends to be a rather simplistic matter. To satisfy the extreme cases, either you run it or you don't. For the middle ground, the only possible option is the choice you have in the matter of timing. This essentially means that sometimes you run it and sometimes you don't.

Such a set of conditions really does not call for sackcloth and ashes. Total flexibility is not always a universal requirement. I have a friend, for example, who specializes in two things and hunts and fishes for nothing else. He fishes for yellowfin tuna on the fifty-fathom curve in the Gulf of Mexico and shoots doves in Monroe County in the fall. There is never a requirement for him to load up four boxes of number-eight shot for one of his fishing trips, and it never occurs to him to want to try to catch yellowfins when he is in a cornfield two miles east of Tunnel Springs.

The two things he wants to do require different equipment—about as far removed in purpose as equipment can get, actually—but neither collection carries with it any requirement for interchangeability.

I had been transferred into pretty much the same position.

The boat had been built to give me the flexibility to be truly amphibious in the river swamp: to be freed from the problem of what the golfing fraternity chooses to call casual water; to be able to reach hitherto inaccessible areas in times of rising water; and to be able to take advantage of the opportunity to hunt either fall turkeys or two species of ducks, one native and one migratory, that coincidentally occupied the same habitat in December.

No duck on this coast stays in the woods except mallards and wood ducks. Along the Mississippi, because there is so much big water, there are lakes that are big enough to serve as open water that can handle a variety of species. In point of fact, there are areas along the river below Memphis that invalidate anything you may have thought you knew about duck hunting if you happen to have been born along the Gulf or the Atlantic coasts.

There they deal with things like puddle ducks in fifteen feet of water. Fixed blinds that have decoys in front of them from the beginning of the season to the end. Comments like, "Business won't get good until we get sunlight on the decoys." Every kind of duck there is in the book is there except for canvasback, and I have been surprised by this region so much and over so many things that I would not bet you that they don't have these, somewhere. They have all the strange situations that can result, in my opinion, from having thousands of acres of rice fields for ducks to feed on next to thousands of acres of big water where they can go and rest.

Over here on the Gulf, we have a different situation. Here

there are woodies and mallards in the river swamp, and everything else is down in the marshes at the head of the bay.

So the boat was parked next to the shed where its individual boards had been stored before construction, and it was obviously going to stay there throughout the turkey seasons, both spring and fall. I floated down Escambia Creek from time to time in the summer and took the boat down to the mouth of the Mobile River in September and October when the redfish and speckled trout run was on. Other than that, it stayed under the shed.

Living eighty miles from the coast and being a coastal duck hunter means you have to deliberately devote whole days to duck hunting. I do not really consider myself a duck hunter. I am a turkey hunter who hunts ducks on off seasons or on windy days during turkey season, in the same way that I hunt snipe and doves when nothing else is open. Hunting ducks from where I then lived meant I had to deliberately give up a day out of the fall turkey season to go eighty miles south to hunt ducks. There was no opportunity to get up in the morning, look out the window, and see enough bad weather to help make up my mind. As a consequence, I simply abandoned duck hunting altogether, considering the game, in this case, not being worth the candle.

But while the area I lived in during this hiatus may have caused a modification in behavior in one direction, it afforded a unique opportunity in another. It gave me the chance to become a daily turkey hunter for the first time in my life.

Daily turkey hunters come in exactly three sizes: the idle rich or their sons; the calculating poor, who fall into two subclassifications—the irresponsible or the opportunistic; and last of all, the remittance men.

The idle rich and their offspring are the people who busy themselves with estate management or coupon clipping and resemble the people in those novels about life in the English countryside during the first half of the nineteenth century.

People who spend most of their time indulging in one form of enjoyment or another and make a career out of finding pleasant occupations designed to fill up the day.

I say this with no resentment at all, but with the clear understanding that most of these people hold such positions because they selected the proper parents to be born to. Occasionally, a man may break the bank at Monte Carlo, or fill enough inside straights, or buy one of those stocks that positively runs amok, or write the great American paragraph and achieve membership at a later stage in his life, but normally, inclusion in the ranks of the idle rich is a condition that is achieved at birth.

I have a friend who puts it beautifully. He says the very best business for a man to get into is the inheriting business.

The calculating poor are able to hunt every day only if they live by their wits. They need the normal amount of money for food, shelter, and amusement like everyone else, but there are certain instances in which a variety of shortcuts can be utilized to fill these requirements.

Some of the calculating poor are—quite frankly and openly—lazy and irresponsible trash. They exist on unemployment compensation, food stamps, aid to dependent children, all of the normal varieties of the dole, and many of the more imaginative expedients. They have been able to swallow their pride and make no bones about living off a combination of the generosity and indifference of the rest of society.

There are not too many of these. Very few people with surnames other than Jukes or Kallikak are able to so subjugate their pride that they are willing to remain in such a group—but there are some.

Of the second of the two subclasses, the ones who are called opportunistic, there is a full slate. These are the ones who are unwilling to work regularly, but are just as unwilling to be seen publicly standing in the food stamp line. These are the ones who seek out and find the various, ingenious substitutions.

They make a little whiskey. They tend to a few cows. They fiddle around with fish boxes in the river. Many of them have wives who do piecework in one or the other of the garment factories scattered across the rural South, faithfully supporting the family while the oldest daughter keeps the house. Those in the opportunistic group not only originate and accept such a state of affairs, they encourage it.

Because so much of the land in the South is owned by the sons of people who inherited farmland that was bought for $10 an acre, many of them sell a little timber from time to time. They have allowed cropland to revert to pasture because they are too trifling to farm, but they can sell timber from what were once the woodlots surrounding the fields.

This group forms the pool from which juries and poll watchers are selected, and they used to be the prime recruiting source for most of the lynch mobs. Any occupation that is irregular in nature, does not require physical exertion, and requires the minimum of intellectual effort is acceptable to them, so long as it does not interfere with hunting and fishing and so long as they can keep the wife working in the shirt factory.

The third and final class of daily hunters is that of the remittance men, a group in which I held an active membership for fifteen years.

The British Empire was the creator of both the term and the occupation. Strictly speaking, a remittance man is someone who is paid a regular stipend to stay away: a younger son who was the family black sheep, a daughter (the term is asexual) who married beneath the family's standards, or a brother who has been guilty of some extremely creative bookkeeping. Someone who is not to be allowed to starve, but whose presence is unwelcome. They are sent sufficient money on a regular basis to allow them to live without creating further scandal, so long as they do not inflict their presence upon the balance of the family. A completely different continent is the usual, preferred location for the degree of separation desired, and normally, the continuation of the stipend is conditional on this distance being maintained.

Among the practitioners of voodoo in sawmills, logging crews, and turpentine camps, there is an interesting subspecies of remittance men. Most of the workers in the forest products industry were not financially able to afford a regular remittance, but they could come up with a single, lump-sum payment when necessary. In return for this payment, the gris-gris or witch lady—called by various names in different locations—would cast a spell upon the subject that was known as the Wandering Foot.

Say, for instance, I became convinced you were paying what I considered to be an undue amount of attention to my wife. Rather than approach you, or her, with the specific accusation, bringing on all the heated discussions such accusations commonly create, I simply went to the local witch doctor and bought your absence.

Properly cast, the spell known as the Wandering Foot made it impossible for you to stay where I was. Unknown pressures caused you to go take a job in another location, or catch the train to Detroit, or decide you had pressing business in Central America, and my problem went away quietly with no questions asked. It precluded having a deputy sheriff coming to the house, wanting to know where I was last Thursday and did anybody see me there—a likely course of events if I was suspected of being one of those people who took personal, corrective action.

I have no idea whether you believe in voodoo or not, and I am indifferent. I neither proselytize nor condemn. I only know that I have seen several instances of just such unexplained absences. I recognize that some of these could have been caused by events not supernatural in nature and that the absence could be permanent. But I do know that some of these witch doctors enjoy repeat business, which means to me that they have, at least, a percentage of satisfied customers.

As a matter of fact, I wish I believed in it myself. I am financially able to come up with the up-front payment and have several likely candidates in mind.

I was not a member of either of these two forms of remittance men. I was a member of the group that is paid to stay away from the offices and do work out in the woods.

Not every woods worker qualifies. Some of them—logging crew members, for example—work in small groups, go to work and leave as a part of that group, are accountable for all hours spent, and the crew is so small that there is not sufficient slack to be able to cover absences.

Timber markers and cruisers (or log scalers) have the option to go early and stay late. What they do with either end of the work day is their own business. Daily hunts may be difficult for these people because they have individual duties that are measurable or have visible results, but they have the option of time. They can hunt before work or after hours, providing that the place where they are working is reasonably close to the area in which they hunt.

People with sufficient rank to direct the actions of others have the most freedom of all. They have no fixed arrival or departure times, no predetermined locations, no specific duties, and are actually required to cover many thousands of acres to properly oversee the people who are their responsibility. If their responsibility is general in nature, then they live in the best of all possible worlds. These last, to be perfectly realistic about it, are the last aristocracy left on earth.

I was promoted out of a job like this some thirty years ago, and it has been downhill every step of the way since.

As a practicing remittance man, and as one who only directed the actions of other people, I was able to hunt every day. With rare exceptions, and those mostly caused by severe weather or high-ranking visitors, I was usually able to hunt every afternoon as well as every morning in the spring.

Any remittance man who hunts this much as a usual thing is obliged to take the maximum amount of care to keep from rubbing it in.

One of the easiest and most successful ploys to keep things from being too obvious is the practice of changing clothes every day in the woods.

Changing clothes in the woods is not at all uncommon. A lot of logging crew members have a set of oil-soaked clothes they wear while running the skidder. Timber markers will have a pair of pants and a shirt that have been spattered so much they become nearly painted, and they wear these only while actively marking. A lot of people go and come in a better-looking set of clothes than they use while wading muddy swamps. There is no chance to take a cold shower in the woods after you finish work, but there is a degree of refreshment to be taken from driving back home in clean clothes.

The class of remittance men to which I belonged did not change clothes in the woods in the interest of cleanliness. They did it so that everybody in town would not see them leaving every morning and coming back every night after dark wearing hunting clothes. They could go out in khakis and switch to camouflage after they got out of the car. Coming back after dark was not as critical as leaving, unless you had to make a stop on the way home, but it never hurt to play it safe. No one ever knew when he might stumble over a broken-down log truck along the way that was his responsibility, and he would have to stop and render assistance.

A remittance man of this group is on the other end of the curve from those clods who cannot resist driving through town with a deer in the back of the pickup. Since cars began to be made with inline fenders, no one ties a deer over the hood as Hunter's Exhibit I anymore, because the heat of the engine can spoil the meat while the trophy is being shown off.

Nowadays, they drop the tailgate of the pickup and pull the deer far enough to the rear to make sure the rack of horns protrudes past the back edge of the tailgate when it is down, which gives everybody a good look at the rack while the driver arranges to catch every red light on the courthouse square as he comes through town. Some of them even make more than one circle around the courthouse to make sure they achieve the maximum visibility.

Your dedicated remittance man not only does not exhibit anything he may have happened to shoot, he takes great pains to hide it. Almost without exception, he tries to give the impression that he only manages to go hunting on alternate Thursdays in alternate Aprils; usually has time to stay no more than thirty minutes even then; and to the best of his recollection, the last turkey he killed was a twelve-pound yearling gobbler, shot out of a chufa patch in the afternoon in March of 1957.

Almost invariably, the remittance man hunts alone. He has arranged his business to free up enough of his time to carry off absences for himself, but it is difficult to have enough clout to free up another person to go along. Even if he can do this, he almost never does, because it is the rarest thing in the world to see them travel in pairs.

Dickens uses a marvelous line in *A Christmas Carol.* He says, in describing Scrooge's entry into his house on Christmas Eve, "Darkness was cheap, and Scrooge liked it."

Being a remittance man is not particularly cheap, but it is solitary, and they like it.

There is a pronounced difference between being solitary and being lonesome. Being solitary means you can quit and go home when it pleases you. You can hunt in any direction you choose and change directions in the middle if you please. On the river you can change a turkey hunt into a duck hunt, or vice versa, without a protracted session of discussions. And you never, ever have to revisit a decision or apologize for an incorrect one.

Being a sole proprietor as a remittance man built in a principal advantage that I did not recognize at the time because I had no expectation of what was coming: It left me free to devote my entire time to the Colonel's daughter and her education, after she got here and got old enough to go.

There was no regular companion I had to work her in with. There was none of the stress that sometimes arises when two people have comfortably hunted together for years and there is suddenly thrown into the pot a third person—not a blood relative of one of the pair—in the form of a lively, active, opinionated child with a vivid imagination and a high-pitched voice.

People handle this all the time, but that is where the rub comes: in the fact that it must be handled.

There is no pleasure in hunting to match that of introducing a young person to the entire experience, so long as you can devote yourself wholly to that person. If the concentration upon that youngster creates a strain, inhibits the actions of anyone at all (either the new member of the group or one of the others), then a great deal of the pleasure is adulterated.

Whatever else that being a long-time remittance man may have caused me to miss in companionship, it left me free to wallow in the pure enjoyment of the company of the Colonel's daughter.

Its second principal advantage was that it showed me the benefits to be gained by hunting every day, an advantage that superceded all others in value.

Bedford Forrest, who had twenty-nine horses shot from under him in various campaigns, kept score. He kept up with the corresponding number of personal successes he enjoyed in the other direction and was the one who first said that he was, "A horse ahead at the close."

The luck of the draw gave me more opportunity than it gave General Forrest because by the time I got back to the river, I was at least two horses ahead.

10

The River System

LTHOUGH YOU AND EVERYBODY ELSE who stands on the bank today would look at it and call it a river, what you really are seeing is something that is not so much a body of water as it is a road. And not only that, but a thing that has been recognized as a road all the way back to prehistoric times.

It is inconceivable to me that the American Indian did not come to realize the principle of the wheel. He had the circular shield. He understood the hoop because he used it in some of his games. He may not have had the potter's wheel as such, but he created pottery on a turntable. There is no way it would never have occurred to him to go the rest of the way and use two circles with a stick joining them at their centers for the axle.

But a wheel is one of those inventions that cannot be used singly. To be properly effective and completely useful, the wheel needs a smooth surface to run on. When you got away from the plains of middle America, this meant that you had to have a road.

The American Indian did not need to go to the trouble to create a road in most of North America because one came with the territory. It was called a stream, and there was one running in almost any direction he wanted to go.

Not only did they run all over the country, but in half the cases, he had the current helping him. He only had to muscle his way along if where he wanted to go happened to be upstream.

So what it really amounted to was that the American Indian didn't develop the wheel because he didn't need one.

All the early transportation systems in the United States were on the water. Rivers were free. Rivers required no extensive labor force to make a roadbed, no maintenance was necessary, and there was no right-of-way to buy. It was easier then to build the town at the edge of the transportation system than it was to construct a transportation system to each of the towns.

It was sort of like what happened when a prehistoric eastern Indian killed a moose with an atl-atl. Because he had no pack animals, and because a fifteen-hundred-pound moose is too heavy to move, he simply went home and walked in the door with the statement, "Pack up. I just killed a moose." They packed, and the whole family moved out to the site of the kill and stayed there until they ate it.

You go where the weight is.

In south Alabama we don't have any white birch with which to build canoes. There were rafts of logs and lumber, and after that there were flatboats and keelboats. Then, beginning in 1818, there was the steamboat.

No matter what it said in your fourth-grade history book, the steamboat was not invented by Robert Fulton in 1807.

In 1790, a man named John Fitch ran a steamboat up and down the Delaware River from Philadelphia to Trenton carrying paying passengers. The boat was in regular operation all during the summer of 1790, seventeen years before Fulton.

Philadelphians, as pointed out years later by W. C. Fields, are not a people prone to take risks. They considered Fitch's invention to be entirely too dangerous and stuck with their old-fashioned stagecoaches. This made Mr. Fitch's boat line lose money, and he eventually abandoned it.

Robert Fulton, in addition to being an inventive type, understood the principles of marketing, had friends in high places, understood the value of advertising and customer relations, came on the scene to take up the slack, made all the money, and got all the ink.

In any event, the steamboat worked its way down the Ohio, got to the Mississippi about 1812 or so, and had gotten over as far as south Alabama by 1818.

The century from 1815 to 1915 very roughly covered the

flush days of steamboating in the United States. While the boats on the Alabama and Tombigbee river systems never reached the peak of splendor achieved either on the Mississippi or in the Northeast, they were nothing to be ashamed of.

When the *Eliza Battle* burned in March 1858 at Myrtlewood on the Tombigbee River, a copy of the manifest shows the boat had on board two hundred passengers, two thousand bales of cotton, two brass bands, and a steam calliope—a collection of equipment substantially beyond that found on an average working flatboat.

The *Aramanth*, which ran the Alabama River in the 1840s, had a third-deck main saloon two hundred feet long with eight cut-glass chandeliers down the middle.

Passage on either of these two vessels hardly constituted roughing it, and even though there was something called deck passage (which meant, in effect, that you sat topside and ate baloney sandwiches), cabin passage river travel in Alabama in those days was directly synonymous with luxury.

The definitive description of a nineteenth-century steamboat was written by a young newspaper reporter named Clyde Fitch who said:

> The steamboat is an engine on a raft, with $11,000 worth of scroll saw work around it.
>
> Steamships are built of steel and are severely plain except on the inside where the millionaire tourists sit. Steamboats are built of wood, tin, shingles, canvas and twine and look like a bride of Babylon. If a steamboat should go to sea, the ocean would take one playful slap at it and people would be picking up kindling on the beach for the next eleven years.
>
> However, the steamboat does not go to sea. Its home is on the river, which does not rise up and stand on end in a storm. It is necessary that a steamboat shall be light and airy because if it were heavy it would stick to the bottom of the river and become an island instead of a means of transportation.
>
> The steamboat is from forty to seventy feet high above the water, but does not extend more than three feet down into the water. This is because that is all the water there is. A steamboat must be built so that when the river is low and the sandbars come out for air, the first mate can tap a keg of beer and run the boat four miles on the suds.

Don't let the low numbers fool you. This was written in a day when $11,000 would buy a township of land.

Railroads began to eat into the business some, about the time of the Civil War, but they did it on the basis of speed. Trains ran forty-five miles an hour rather than fifteen, and the fact was that they went into places where there were no rivers to float steamboats.

But for pure swank, for the opportunity to cut yourself a slice of kid-glove, diamond stick-pin, solid-gold, conspicuous consumption, the steamboat was the only game in town. Floating was the only way to go, and in lower Alabama you floated on the *Aramanth* or the *Nettie Quill* or the *Eliza Battle.*

From Mobile to Montgomery on the Alabama River is a distance of 250 miles. There were sixty-four named landings between the two towns, and at almost all of them was someone in attendance day and night. They were there either to load or unload any combination of cargo and passengers or to serve as wood yard attendants, because steamboats, until nearly the very end, burned wood for fuel.

These rivers were as busy in the nineteenth century as the interstate highway system is today. But the roadsides, the lands on both sides of the river between the landings, were pretty much a solitude. Two things kept them that way: the yearly floods and the nature of the timber.

For the first thirty miles upstream from the mouth of the two rivers in Alabama, the land on both sides is what is called blackwater river swamp. The soil is extremely rich, it accretes rather than erodes, and it is renewed yearly by a fresh load of alluvial soil deposited by the annual floods. The water table is no more than eighteen inches under the surface, and the action of the tides (tides are felt as far as thirty miles upstream) brings the water table nearly to the surface on every high tide. As a consequence, both the aerobic and the anaerobic bacteria in the soil get the maximum benefit from water conditions, and the decomposition rate in the soil—a measurement indicative of soil fertility—is as high as that of any place in the world. It would grow the hell out of crops except for two things: At high tide, the water table is six inches under the surface; and in most years, for periods of time during floods that last as long as three consecutive months, the land becomes the bottom of a lake.

Most hardwood trees, unlike conifers, can withstand periods of flooding. With only a few exceptions, they can take it for protracted periods of time, so all the timber along the rivers is composed of hardwood with a very little bit of cypress.

The lower part of the river, the blackwater swamp portion, will go under four or five feet of water during these floods.

The part north of that, what is called the red river swamp portion, has far deeper water. Low water at Coffeeville on the Tombigbee will be eighteen feet—the flood of 1961 had a reading of sixty-one feet at that point. But as far as crops are concerned, a two-foot flood is as deadly as twenty, which means that all the farmlands seen by people like Romans, Taitt, and Bartram along the lower river systems when they visited here just after the American Revolution had been flooded out of business by the time the steamboats got here in 1815.

Before 1840, if you couldn't farm it, you didn't want it, and losing a crop to the flood three years out of four meant you couldn't farm it, or at least you didn't have to. There was cultivatable land going begging two miles away from the river, and anybody who wanted to farm could go there.

What little timber business there was before 1850 was all softwood and all for local consumption except for cypress. River swamp timber, which was all hardwood, came in nothing but the larger sizes and wouldn't float when the wood was green, so nobody was dumb enough to go into the swamp and fool with four-foot-diameter hardwood that was too big to saw after you broke your ass trying to cut it down with axes. (It had to be cut with axes—the invention of the crosscut saw was still thirty years in the future.)

By the time the steamboat business dried up and went away in 1915, the logging industry was in full swing, but it concerned itself with logging longleaf pine on dry ground and moving the timber by railroad. As a consequence, during the half-century from 1915 to 1965, the river swamp in essence became the land that God forgot.

There was a modest amount of hardwood lumber made and sold, but it came from only the finest trees. What little logging going on was done with pull boats and cables, and pull-boat logging (which featured logs dragged to the bank of the river by cables on steam-driven drums) is slow, hard, and expensive. The lack of markets for lower grades and poorer species led to a very limited hardwood logging industry and a system of logging known as diameter-limit cutting. Diameter-limit logging is the current euphemism for high grading.

Take passenger service off the rivers, to such an extent that sixty-four landings in 250 miles become fewer than two dozen, with all those remaining serving only as boat-launching facilities for fishermen (as happened in 1915); transfer all freight to the railroads beyond that of a few barge loads of hardwood logs of steadily decreasing quality; abandon virtually all farming because of the danger of recurring floods; and a river will die on your hands.

Compared with 1875, the rivers of Alabama in 1965 were like those ghostly mining towns in the far West that consist of a single street of vacant, dilapidated buildings where there were formerly seven saloons, two general stores, a bank, an opera house, and two stagecoaches a day. The only thing the present town has left is the name.

Rivers undergoing aggradation in a lower flood plain sometimes commit suicide over part of their length by cutting through the neck of a bend at high water and leaving what is called an oxbow lake to fill in over the years. Parts of rivers can be killed by governmental agencies. This happened on the Alabama in the case of the Fort Mims cutoff, where a cut of a trifle more than a mile, from Wilkin Bend across the top of Hogan's Bend, shortened the river by ten miles, made two islands with a combined area of some two thousand acres, and left both Montgomery Hill Landing and Pierce's Landing thrown away and abandoned out in the woods on a dead lake.

In the eight miles above the junction of the Alabama and the Tombigbee, there are nine such killings and suicides still visible on the U.S. Geological Survey maps. If you take a look at aerial photographs of the same area, which lets you pick out those oxbow lakes too old and small to appear on the contour map, you will also see some that are so ancient they have become nothing but meander scars. You get an appreciation of how much of the swamp is water, even with the rivers not in flood.

What you had left—after the demise of transportation, the abandonment of farming, the lack of roads because of the terrain, and the absence of a logging industry—was a part of the state with a principal value of keeping the sunlight out of hell. From the standpoint of those of us who hunt and fish, this was a consummation devoutly to be wished.

By 1925, the last of the old-growth pine had been cut. Millions of acres in the state consisted of rolling hillsides of blackjack oak interspersed with two cords of pine per acre. Eroded and abandoned farms were sending thousands of tons of topsoil each year into the Gulf of Mexico. Deer were reduced nearly to the point of extinction, and turkeys lived mainly as characters in the lies told by old men to one another.

The 2.3 million acres of bottomland hardwood in the river swamp (ten percent of the forested area of the state)—the lands that nobody wanted—are what brought fish and game back into the sunlight.

They were the yeast that raised the bread.

This is why so many of us old crocks who remember what things were like have such a love affair with river swamplands. We are aware of what they have done, we know how much we all owe to them, and we remember who held the fort when everything else was either abandoned farms or two cords of pine per acre scattered across a sea of scrub oak.

The lands are not the swamp as depicted by Hollywood, with everybody in waist-deep water swinging his machete at the vines and a crocodile under every bush, but there is enough water in sufficient depth at nearly every stage of the river to call itself to your attention and cause you to make arrangements to deal with it.

Down here, these bodies of water—be they sloughs, runs, guts, lakes, ponds, or streams—never freeze over with sufficient ice to let you walk across them. I saw a photograph the other day with an article pointing out that the track event of pole vaulting was a part of the ancient Taileaan Games in Ireland. It is still in use in Holland by farmers to cross drainage ditches in their fields, but is intended to achieve distance rather than height. The article was absorbingly interesting, but there is still a question or two in my mind about using pole vaulting here.

Can you put the butt of the pole in the middle of the water and, if so, how firm does the bottom of the body of water have to be?

Is there a chance that the vaulting pole would begin to sink as you approached the apogee of your vault, preventing you from crossing over and letting you slowly lean either to port or starboard until you got wet? Or worse, would you sink so quickly that you are left stranded in the middle, clutching your pole like a monkey on a stick, with only the option of climbing what pole you have left above you while you sink inexorably into the waiting water?

If you happen to be a direct lineal descendant of Moses and have inherited his rod, then you need no help at all in stream crossings and these paragraphs are unnecessary.

If you are one of the plain people, have neither a rod to part the waters nor the gymnastic ability to vault stream crossings in a single bound, and are too candy-assed to simply wade through anything less than neck-deep, there remains a dull, uninspired, plain-vanilla solution.

Get yourself a small boat like the rest of us clods, and leave it in the swamp where you are going to use it.

Like so many other things in the world, this *speaks* a hell of a lot easier than it *does*. In fact, as soon as you decide to do it, you open the same Pandora's box the rest of us have been struggling with all these years.

Where the hell do you leave the boat, because how do you know before the fact where you will be when you want it?

A few of the available options are easy. If you are simply using it to cross the river or to change locations on the river, then you leave it on the trailer and tow it from place to place.

If you hunt ducks on one lake or in one particular maze of sloughs, then you can leave it at the point where you normally enter this particular region and walk to it to start.

If you fish in the spring in one particular place, it becomes a knee-slapper. In such a case, you can even build a rack on the side of the lake to leave it on when you are not using it.

The trouble comes when you have to decide where you want to leave it when you are engaged in the matter of crossing various bodies of water and are not really interested in the water itself—other than the fact that it constitutes an obstacle—but in what is happening on the other side.

The old lady fortune-tellers in my family, who told fortunes mostly with cards, were always talking about how the cards saw a package coming to the house, from across the water, carried by a dark man.

It is those areas across the water, where the packages come from, that will require most of your ingenuity and creativity and will create the most opportunity for you to make lightning decisions.

This can get pretty complicated because of the nature of rivers in flat country. For example, when the river stage at Claiborne, a station on the Alabama River, gets up to twenty feet, it has a pronounced effect upon a place I hunt that is forty miles downstream.

There is a dip in the road there, just past the pine hills, that turns from a low place in the road into a creek nearly forty feet wide, waist-deep in the middle, and with a four-knot current. Behind this crossing, which is then a ford with a rock bottom, is an area of nearly three thousand acres that are sealed off here, because the stage of the river is up to twenty feet at a place forty miles to the north.

There are other watery areas in these three thousand acres that have activity going on across them. If the boat is left at the first crossing, the only thing you have gained is that you can get over the first forty feet with dry legs, assuming the current is not too swift to paddle through, and you then have 2998.8 acres in front of you with no boat to use on any of them.

I have given a single example. There are almost as many possibilities as there are acres, and you cannot cover all the bases before the fact.

The answer, obviously, is more than one boat. But where does the size of the fleet stop? Leaving multiple boats in the swamp is a many-faceted solution for a reason beyond the number of boats, because you must then be able to forecast both ends of the flood.

At some point in the fall, you have to go gather them all up. Later on, after you have decided there will be no more high water, you have to go put them all back in.

If you were a person of unlimited finances, you could afford some two dozen boats, located at strategic points of your selection. You would have to have sufficient funds available to hire a half dozen helpers to get everything out before the water came up in the winter and put everything back after the floods left in the spring. Having unlimited people would not be of any help in forecasting these floods, but you could evade forecasting altogether if you were rich enough to have all your boats put out in the morning and taken in at dark every day, like the flag.

This, of course, is fantasy. It's the equivalent of asking Santa Claus to leave you 250 duck decoys and two men to set them out and take them up.

Once, years ago, I was in charge of an experimental logging operation that used skids and pallets. Trees were cut down, cut into six-foot lengths, and loaded into racks—called pallets—that held about two cords of wood each. These were skidded to the side of the road after loading, winched up on a truck, and hauled to the mill.

We had, as I recall it, between fifty and sixty pallets.

It wouldn't have made a particle of difference if we had had five hundred.

Sooner or later, the world being the kind of place that it is, all the pallets on hand would be full, all the empties would be at some point four miles away, both haul trucks would be fifty miles away and going in the opposite direction, and the entire operation would turn up its toes and die in place.

I will never have an opportunity to find out for sure, but I am willing to be positive about the fact that if you had two dozen boats, four boat movers, unlimited financial resources, and total communications between all interested parties, there would be days when you would be nailed behind impossible obstacles and there would be times when you got a wet ass just finding out that the obstacles were impossible.

The best probable solution is to have two boats (one to drive from place to place and one to leave in the swamp), a modest amount of brains, an open mind, and a willingness to discover field expedients.

11

Field Expedients

JOHN C. HOLMAN of the 117th Artillery was promoted to captain during the Louisiana maneuvers in 1940. Dwight D. Eisenhower was a participant in the same maneuver at the same time, but at that time held the rank of lieutenant colonel.

John made major in 1959, by which time Lt. Col. Eisenhower had been promoted six times, had held every rank in the army above lieutenant colonel (including five star general), had won two national elections, and was then serving his second term as president of the United States.

In John's defense, he had been promoted to major in Korea in 1953. Under the ground rules in operation at the time, however, the Alabama National Guard did not recognize promotions awarded on active duty, and an individual reverted to the rank he had held in the guard when he got back from active duty.

Leaving out this brief hiccup in the flow, which was the equivalent of what baseball players would describe as "having a cup of coffee as a major," John Holman remained a captain for nineteen years.

You should not take any of this to mean that Dwight Eisenhower was all that much smarter than John Holman or all that much better a soldier either. There is always some element of chance in whatever promotions happen to befall us, and it is never a matter of pure justice that causes these things to happen exactly as we deserve them.

John was, of course, aware of the difference in time span between the speed of his promotions and the speed of those of the incumbent president in 1959, but was in no sense discouraged by it. He considered it to have no bearing on the main business at hand.

He was a member of that class of Americans that Emerson called the "embattled farmers," the descendants of the ones who stood at the rude bridge at Concord and have been, figuratively, standing at a succession of rude bridges in the service of the United States ever since.

John was among the kind of people W. H. Auden had in mind when he wrote the lines: "When there was peace, he was for peace. When there was war, he went."

John began his career as a horse holder in C Battery of the 117th in 1926. He fought and was decorated in two wars and was retired as a major, finally, from headquarters of the same battalion in 1967, forty-one years after he had first enlisted.

Professional members of the Embattled Farmers Association concern themselves with tending to the business of the United States in time of war. They spend little time agonizing over the relatively rapid promotions enjoyed by members of the Regular Establishment.

And it was John Holman, when he and I were standing at one of those rude bridges together one afternoon, who gave me the clearest possible example of what the army means when it talks about a "field expedient."

A field expedient is the action you take when, rather than complaining that you were not issued the proper equipment and resources for the job at hand, you press on and effect a solution with what you do have. New Englanders call it "making do."

The year was 1951 and Captain John at that time had only been in grade for ten years, a period of time, as it turned out, hardly long enough for the new to have worn off. A series of transfers, schools, assignments to other units, and formations of cadres had left the battalion horribly short of officers; short to the point that I had been given command of A Battery as a second lieutenant with five months service. That assignment brings to mind John Randolph's comment on John Quincy Adams's selection of one of his cabinet members, that "never were abilities so much below mediocrity so well rewarded. Not even when

Caligula's horse was made consul of Rome." But at any rate, the assignment had been made; a battery in those days was composed of ninety-six men, eight officers, and four cannon; and I was the little child who led them.

Someone up the line in division artillery with nothing more worthwhile available to fill up his time one dull afternoon had promulgated the edict that all officers would produce whatever paperwork they had to substantiate the decorations to which they were entitled. The ribbons of such decorations were to be worn during duty hours.

Battalion headquarters, with its tongue firmly in its cheek, had passed this edict down, and people patiently hunted through whatever paperwork they had available to come up with sufficient data to certify their ribbons.

At the battery commanders meeting that afternoon, I happened to sit next to Captain John. In shifting things from one hand to the other, he dropped several pieces of paper on the planer mill shavings that floored the Colonel's tent. I was helping him pick them up, when right in the middle of all this the Colonel asked him a question. When John stopped to answer, I finished picking up, and while he was still talking to the Colonel and I was waiting for him to finish, I looked down at the top document I had picked up and had not yet handed over.

The paper was a citation, written in French. It had been folded across in half and then across again into quarters and had penciled notes on the back of one of the folds.

There was no date but there was a note that was headed, "B. C. Meeting 1600." The first entry written was, "Do we have any condoms?"

The document was the citation that accompanied the award of the Croix de Guerre.

I did not read French then, don't now as a matter of fact, but I could puzzle out a word or two. His name was clearly entered as the recipient of the award, and I know enough French to know what the Croix de Guerre is.

I am aware that gentlemen do not read each other's mail and can only defend my actions upon the basis of surprise and the fact that this paper was right on top. I had seen a ribbon in his set of decorations that I did not recognize, the last ribbon in the last row, a green one that had four narrow, red, vertical stripes. I was aware that ribbons denoting foreign decorations are worn last, but did not realize that this meant last even behind the "I was there" ribbons of the United States. Nor did I consider myself to be an expert on foreign decorations and awards.

But the Croix de Guerre is awarded only for bravery, can come only from the French government, and the citation for such an award is surely deserving of more respect than to have been folded twice and used as notepaper. Moreover, notepaper used to record what appeared to me to be entirely inappropriate material.

I remember thinking that it was a blessing this man had not been present at the ceremony held at the grave of Lafayette in Paris at the beginning of World War I. Rather than making the comment that General Pershing offered on behalf of the American army at the time, "LaFayette, we are here," this man would have been likely to paraphrase General Sheridan's comment on Indians and say, "The only good Frog is a dead Frog."

I made, of course, no comment at the time. Five-month-service second lieutenants with any sense of self-preservation at all do not question extremely senior captains. But I am cursed in having one of those unfortunate faces that do a wholly inferior job of hiding the thoughts that are going through the head behind the face.

I have had it called to my attention many times in the years since then that my thoughts are so obvious I might as well wear a sign and, obviously, Captain John caught the expression. As we left the Colonel's tent after the meeting, he told me that the decoration had been awarded, complete with a kiss on each cheek, at a battalion formation in France, and that after the formation and the departure of the decorating contingent, there had been a quick battery commanders meeting.

Caught without his notebook, he had to write on whatever paper he had, and he felt it would look less ostentatious if he folded the citation into quarters before he wrote on the back. He said he intended to get it framed later, in which case the back would not show, but had never gotten around to it. It had simply been a matter of necessity. There was no intention to insult every soldier the French nation had produced nor to demean every decoration they had awarded since the time of Charlemagne. He was only making do with what he had.

I cannot remember what I said when he finished. It must have been inadequate and inane, but in the forty-five years that have passed since the incident, I have been able to think of no bright, clever remark whatsoever that I should have made in apology for my unkind thoughts.

The lesson, however, struck home. I have carefully refrained from bitching about my lack of equipment on almost every occasion since. In point of fact, I have gone nearly too far in the other direction several times. Like the time I told the major general that it was a matter of complete indifference to me that we had been issued no camouflage netting to hide the howitzers— that we intended to build brush arbors over them, like people used to use at old-fashioned revivals, which would not only hide the guns but could conceivably establish a climate that would encourage the cannoneers to sing hymns between fire missions.

The kind of remark, now that I come to think about it, that may have helped me to remain a captain for nearly ten years myself.

It is these pointed examples you are shown when you are still young that do so much to educate you and that you find yourself using in later years, especially if the examples come from a person whose conduct you find admirable. Almost by instinct, you find yourself not complaining about the lack of a piece of equipment. You have become conditioned, like Pavlov's dog.

When it comes to making do with boats, probably the simplest and most straightforward of the water-crossing expedients, after a simple crossing of the river from one side to another, is the situation that arises where a series of sloughs run into the river. In such an instance, it is frequently possible to float the river in the dark, and after turkeys gobble, if they do, land the boat on the proper side of the slough and go to the turkey from there.

A turkey exhibits a remarkable reluctance to cross water himself. He may roost over it through preference, and frequently does, and he may gobble from that watery roost at some length. Nor is it at all unusual for him to fly more than a hundred yards when he comes off the roost, and it does not appear to bother him if the flying portion of the dismount happens to be over the water. But once he is down, once he begins to gobble on the ground, he has chosen his side of the water, and most of the time he will stay on that side. Quite often he will come to the edge of the water and walk back and forth, gobbling some, strutting some, putting his best effort into appearing both vocal and decorative, but only on his side of the water. He expects you to come to him.

There are occasions where you can't get to his side for any one of a hundred reasons and are forced into the position of getting to the edge, calling him to a point across the slough, shooting him there, and handling the retrieve in whatever way seems best after the fact; swimming, wading, finding a log, going back for the boat, or whatever.

Such a course of action really ought to be considered only in the final resort category because so many bad things can happen after the shot. The worst-case scenario of all is to have him flop into the slough in his death throes and float downstream, leaving you to run along the bank on your side, simultaneously trying to keep him in sight, wishing he would float over to your side and trying to figure out a plan of action while on the move.

Floating down the river in the dark, waiting for a turkey to gobble so you can decide which side of the slough you want to land the boat on to go to him, is best done in stretches of the river that are dead—killed either by murder or suicide—and no longer have the hazard of the constant passage of boats and barges.

Boats do not come down the river in the dark. They are accompanied by a world of noise, complete with flashing lights. The tug will pick up your boat on its radar if you are unintelligent enough to run without lights yourself, and the chances of hearing a turkey while the noise and racket of a passing boat is going on are very slim indeed. But a nine-barge tow is thirty-five yards wide and two hundred yards long and makes a good deal of wake, and large recreational boats make even more wake than barges and are not nearly so particular about slowing down.

If you were not careful to pull your boat well up into the slough you proposed to walk down to get to the turkey, but left it exposed and hastily tied to a root on the bank of the river, you have left yourself at risk. There is the very real chance of something coming by on the river while you are in the woods and having its wake swamp your tethered boat.

There are few things so aggravating as to come back to where the boat was tied and see the line stretching down into the water with your swamped boat on the other end of it.

Not only is a sunken boat remarkably heavy to pull up, but an hour or so of total submergence does not do a lot of good things to an outboard motor, and it is astonishing how much impedimenta there is scattered around inside the boat that floats off as it submerges.

Approach marches to turkeys fall generally into three broad categories, the last of which is the final few yards when you are trying to decide how close you dare go and trying to find a decent place to set up. This phase is almost invariably done on foot, and while it hardly ever turns into a sneak, the last ten yards can often be legitimately described as a creep.

The first phase is normally the high-speed phase. It is often handled by vehicle and includes the drive from the camp house to the point where you park and the trip up, down, or across the river or to the other end of the lake to get to the point where you expect to hear the turkey gobble.

It is the middle part—the part between where you hear the original gobble until you get to the place where you intend to sit—that has the most variety of all.

This can be done on foot, by boat, by bicycle, or by some involved and interesting combination of all three. Here is where the ability to do mental broken field running becomes a requirement. This is the part that requires you to not only make decisions very rapidly, but to carry them out very quickly after they are made, and it is the part of the operation that requires you to make the most use of field expedients.

It is in this stage that you are apt to find that the method you used is not the one you would have used if you had known what the situation was going to turn into. It is the point at which you have to take some very rapid half-measures, do some things you would prefer not to do, and accept the fact that it is too late to go back and start over. If it means you have to sit in the middle of the road and try to hide behind a pine cone or back up to a huckleberry bush a half-inch in diameter and two feet high, then you must do it. You can only hope for a wide pine cone, a thick bush, or a turkey with poor eyesight.

Dithering, at this stage, is crippling. But there is something even worse than dithering, and that is the tendency to revisit decisions after they are made.

The penalty for revisiting decisions made in this phase goes beyond crippling and becomes terminal. There is only one proper solution. Pick the most likely expedient from whatever paucity of choices you happen to have at hand and play the cards as dealt.

Nobody ever said it was going to be easy.

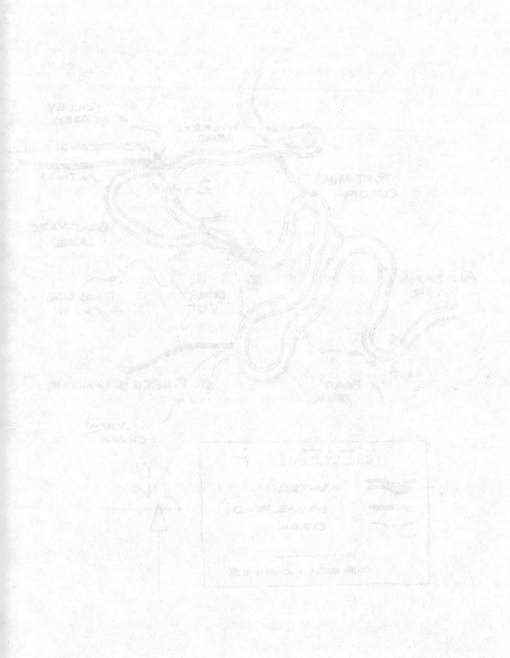

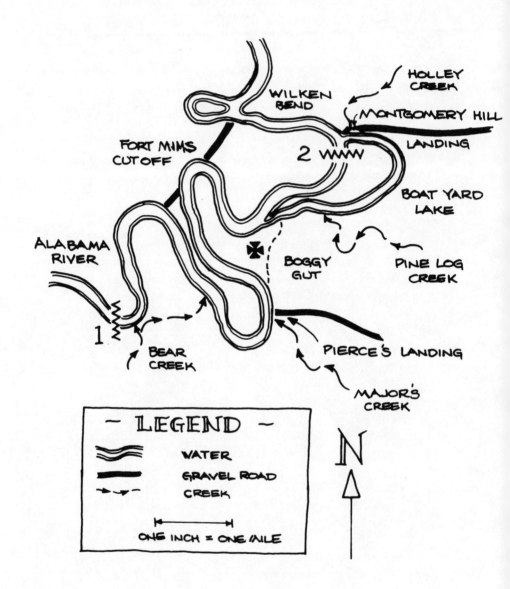

HOLLEY CREEK

WILKEN BEND

MONTGOMERY HILL

LANDING

FORT MIMS CUTOFF

2

BOAT YARD LAKE

ALABAMA RIVER

BOGGY GUT

PINE LOG CREEK

1

BEAR CREEK

PIERCE'S LANDING

MAJOR'S CREEK

- LEGEND -

WATER

GRAVEL ROAD

CREEK

ONE INCH = ONE MILE

N

12

Another
Man's Poison

NOBODY HAS EVER been able to make me comfortable with the existing procedures in handling land mitigation programs or has even been convincing in the explanations as to how the loss of lands can be mitigated. When the Corps of Engineers built the Tenn-Tom Waterway in 1990, whatever you may or may not think of the value of the project, they necessarily had to do some dredging, straighten out some curves, cut through some bends, and otherwise turn several thousands of acres of what was formerly dry land into water.

Not only land, but mostly bottomland hardwood timberland, the type that produces much more game food and that consequently should be able to carry more game per acre than the usual mixed stand of pine and hardwood in the uplands.

Flooding bottomland hardwood makes for more fish because it makes more standing water. Because dams are usually built in such projects, presumably there is opportunity to generate more power. There are instances in which these projects assure the source of water for large segments of the population, and sometimes the purpose of the project is to improve navigation. But no matter what is highest on your list of priorities—fishing, getting more electricity at cheaper cost, having water to irrigate your corn, or having a place to sail your boat—there is no question but that part of the land, what the Bible calls the firmament, has now been permanently turned into the bottom of a lake.

There are certain instances in which such a transition is

clearly in the public interest, and if this is so, then there is no doubt that turning that particular piece of land into the bottom of a lake is using the land for the highest and best use for the most people in the long run.

I do not question such use, although irrigating deserts in order to make them wet enough to grow rice is a little far out on the lunatic fringe, even for Californians. But the thing I have the most problem with is that bred-in-the-bone feeling held by a large part of our population that the losses of these lands can be mitigated—"mitigation" being the current eco-speak definition for replacement.

In the last few years, a corporation near my home sold nearly twenty thousand acres to the Corps of Engineers as mitigation lands to replace those lands turned into lake bottoms by the Tenn-Tom Waterway.

There was no pressure put on anybody from either side. It was a textbook example of a willing seller and a willing buyer getting together.

The lands sold as mitigation lands were bottomland hardwood types, were in an area along the construction site of the waterway, and were all down at one end of the project, of course—but you can't have everything. It is unreasonable to expect to be able to buy land back in every case immediately adjacent to where you flooded other lands, and the price paid was fair to both sides.

Nobody ripped off the dumb-ass government, and no overpowering and ruthless bureaucracy trampled on the rights of private citizens.

Everybody ought to be happy.

The Corps has satisfied the requirement that lands affected by the construction of the waterway be mitigated.

Those members of the environmental community way out at the end of the bell curve can take a great deal of satisfaction over the fact that twenty thousand acres have come back into the public domain and that they have now become entitled to exercise their yeasty imaginations on the management of such lands.

But no matter how hard you strain, no matter how many adjectives you scatter throughout the press announcement, no matter how many arms are sprained by people patting themselves on the back taking credit for the whole thing, the same twenty thousand acres of bottomland hardwood that existed before the sale still exist. They are simply held under different ownership.

It no longer belongs to the corporation; it now belongs to the federal government. The lands drowned in the construction of the waterway remain just as drowned as they were before they became officially mitigated.

The emperor is exactly as naked as he was before.

There are two major losers. The county in which the lands are located has lost the ad valorem tax revenue that was paid annually when the owner was a private citizen (federal lands pay no taxes to the state in which they are located), and the timber—formerly grown on the twenty thousand acres that is now a fish farm—is no longer grown because there are twenty thousand acres less bottomland hardwood than there used to be.

There are two winners, one major and one minor.

The first and most numerous of the two winners is that segment of the population that wants all lands to revert back to federal lands because it gives them the same warm feeling you get from a two-hundred-dollar blanket. This is the transition of a major block in that direction. You may say, if you wish, that now the corporation cannot sell the lands to the Japanese who could then turn it into concrete parking lots. You are going to have to stifle your critical sense before you make such a statement, because we both know that no entity, American or Japanese, could get permission to drain and fill such wetlands, and the land will simply remain in the same state it was in before the trade.

So after all the smoke has cleared, the county has lost whatever amount of the tax money the lands brought in. The drowned lands remain drowned. The amount of land in bottomland hardwood types has been reduced by twenty thousand acres, the acreage of land in lake bottoms has been increased by the same amount, but the world has been made a better place for fish and sailboats.

There is one minor winner. A winner in the persons of the members of a strange subculture that benefits in a strange way.

They are a few turkey hunters who, believe it or not, had nothing to do with the trade, whose wishes were not consulted, and who benefit in a way that reverses an aphorism. For in this instance, one man's poison has truly become another man's meat.

I have the good fortune to be included in this favored group of those who have been rewarded through fallout—at least on this one occasion.

Military historians invariably find it necessary to include tactical maps of troop dispositions and terrain when they come to write about various engagements. People with no appreciation of maps sometimes find this proclivity annoying, but by and large, there is little chance of clarity without it. While this mitigation is not a tactical engagement, it is a discussion of an area where more than one thing goes on, and the reference map on page 96 is almost a necessity in order to have any chance of getting the thought across at all.

The map is of an area of some twenty-five square miles. It is a portion of the Alabama River near Ft. Mims Cutoff. The scale is one inch to the mile, and the area thus covered is roughly sixteen thousand acres. The flow of the river at this point is northeast to southwest, with variations, and the Maltese cross in the center of the map, near the words Boggy Gut, does not designate the location of treasure, but rather where turkeys have been prone to gobble regularly every spring for the past forty years.

Until 1968, the dashed lines in the northwest part of the area—those labeled Ft. Mims Cutoff—were simply lines on the proposed plan of the cutoff in somebody's office at the U.S. Army Corps of Engineers. Tugboats running the Alabama River followed the main course of the river. A person sitting at the Maltese cross could hear the boat's engines from the zigzag line in the southwest corner of the map, near the number 1, to the zigzag line near the number 2, just below Montgomery Hill Landing in the upper-right-hand corner—a distance by river of almost ten miles. At no point along that ten-mile stretch of river would the boat be more than a mile and a half from a person located near the Maltese cross, and along most of that distance, it would be within a mile of him.

Tugboats pushing barges on a river as small as this one run at a speed of five miles per hour. When the Alabama is bank-full, when it is just about to come out of its banks in the yearly flood, the current is at its strongest, and an upstream boat is liable to make less speed than that. A downstream boat, faced with the necessity to flank both the bend above and the bend below the Maltese cross, is not going to average five miles an hour either.

What all this means is that if a turkey has gobbled at daylight, just as a tug has come into hearing at either end of the ten-mile stretch between the two zigzag lines you see on the map, a hunter is going to be faced with the necessity of trying to work his way to that turkey, then trying to work him to his call, over the noise of diesel engines that will sometimes sound as if they are right under his elbow. And they are going to be right there for the next two hours.

It is a perfect example of the fact that two hours can sometimes seem like a week and a half.

I used to leave the boat at the point where the road comes down to Pierce's Landing. Neither Boggy Gut on the north nor Major's Creek on the south can be forded on foot. Boggy Gut is only waist deep in the middle, but it is not called boggy for nothing. Waist-deep water with a bottom that lets you sink another two feet takes every bit of the bloom right off the rose and puts water on the Adam's apple to boot. The water at the mouth of Major's Creek is nearly ten feet deep, and unless you are equipped with lead shoes and don't have to breathe a lot, you can't wade there either. The boat, fulfilling the purpose for which is was built, left you independent of both water depth and bottom conditions at either place.

A boat put in the river at Pierce's Landing gives access to the area north of Boggy Gut, the area south of Major's Creek, and the area directly across the river. In none of the above instances does it require a paddle of more than two hundred yards.

It isn't even necessary to leave the boat at the river bank itself. It can be left a hundred yards up in Boggy Gut or Major's Creek, making it invisible to casual traffic on the river, and worked from there to any point in almost the same time frames. The hundred yards lost on one end is gained on the other.

But in the boat or out of it, you have to put up with the noise.

Tugboat engine noises are nothing like the racket made by jet aircraft, or even the noise made by logging skidders as they were sold before the Occupational Safety and Health Administration regulations on allowable decibel levels.

But then, a turkey does not rank up there with a buffalo stampede so far as noise is concerned either.

Turkey noises are subtle, require both experience and concentration to make anything out of, and, while they may be plain to the experienced ear, do not overpower competition very well.

The worst possible combination of circumstances was to hear a turkey gobble at about the Maltese cross, use the boat to get north across Boggy Gut, and just about the time you got out of the boat on the north side of the Gut hear an upstream-bound boat come around the second bend north of the river's junction with the Tombigbee and get level with Bear Creek slough on the Alabama.

The river at that point—and for the next mile—runs due north, and the sound stays at the intensity it had when you first heard it for just about the length of time it takes for you to get to the turkey and get set up. After the boat rounds this right-hand bend and turns southeast, it has to run a mile and three quarters to get below you to an abrupt left-hand turn that sends it back northwest. At this point, when the boat passes you in the river, the engine sounds as loud as it would if you were standing on the deck of the vessel itself. It goes out to the end of the penin-sula that forms Hogan's Bend, turns right around and comes back, and when it comes level with the entrance to Boatyard Lake, it is about as close to you again as it was forty minutes ago when it first went by.

At this stage, you have heard nothing but boat noises for nearly an hour; you have no idea if the turkey heard anything you had to say or said anything back; and the whole affair has taken on the surreal aspect you would expect to experience if you had attended a silent movie, had been asked to turn your back to the screen as the speed of the music being played by the piano was varied, and ten minutes later had been asked to re-port what had been happening to the characters while your back was turned.

Ninety-five percent of turkey hunting is conducted by sound. Except for those turkeys that star in videos produced by one of the various call-makers—in which turkeys come to the call in groups of three, gobble every time the caller yelps, and only stop gobbling when the trigger is pulled—a turkey in the real world who comes to your calling is usually silent there at the last. He may have gobbled fifty times, you may have heard him drum-ming or walking in the leaves for thirty minutes, but almost al-ways, just there at the end, before you see him, he stands mute and everything gets quiet.

It is one of the things that puts so much uncertainty in the sport. Have you run him off? Is he standing out there just in range waiting to see the calling hen? If he has not run off, how long is he going to wait before making a noise so you will know where he is? What is the proper length of time for you to suffer in silence before you do something? And what is the thing you ought to do to trigger him into giving you a location (something not completely stupid, that is)?

None of this ought to be conducted to the sound of diesel engines at your elbow. Nobody ought to be given tickets to hear the London Philharmonic and then be forced to sit with ear-phones on, listening to recordings of tank engines being warmed up and taking what pleasure he can from watching the London Philharmonic saw away in silence.

All of which was a very fair approximation of what you found yourself doing very frequently a mile north of Pierce's Landing on the Alabama River in the years before the Corps of Engineers built the Ft. Mims Cutoff.

After the cutoff, boats go directly from the river at Wilkin Bend, touch it again briefly at the end of Hogan's Bend, and then cut across the narrow neck just above Milepost 12 and get back in the river again.

A ten-mile stretch of the river has been abandoned to the backwoods, and at any point along that stretch you can now take off your earphones and listen to the orchestra.

If you are riding the *Nettie Quill* from Wilkin Bend to Mobile, your travel time has been reduced by two hours—except the *Nettie Quill* hasn't run for seventy-five years, and there is no longer a dock at Wilkin Bend to board from.

There is a boat landing at Boatyard Lake and one at the mouth of Holley Creek—both offering public launching, ice, bait, and soft drinks—both now living on borrowed time. The river is filling in the old bed at the upstream end first, but it will eventually seal in the downstream side as well. It will still be possible to get into the river from either boat landing for some time to come, but the handwriting is on the wall for the pair of them, and both establishments will eventually have been sacrificed on the altar of navigational improvement.

Strictly speaking, the Ft. Mims Cutoff is not on the Tombigbee River at all. Consequently, the sixty-one acres of bottomland turned to water by this cutoff was not due to land-use changes caused by the Tenn-Tom project. Mitigation funds were made available to replace any lands in the vicinity, and the Ft. Mims Cutoff qualified under this provision.

The point—if you are willing to concede there is a point at all—is that while land-use changes can sometimes be in the public interest for any of the reasons already covered, it cannot be much stronger than highly questionable that lands that have been flooded can be replaced.

There is an instance of replacement in Mobile Bay. As part of the spoil disposal problem some years ago, an island was created near the western shore of the bay where none existed before. This island serves as a remarkably fine nesting site for several species of birds, prominent among them the brown pelican.

This island is an example of low, wet land being created where none existed before. It has been done at the expense of an area that was in shallow water that could conceivably have produced oyster reefs, thereby changing shallow water into low-lying islands. I am confident that the oystermen in Mobile County are not as ecstatic over the creation of this island as is the Audubon Club.

We live in a round world, and, like the cat in the round house, there are no corners in which to defecate.

The Ft. Mims Cutoff gave back to turkey hunters the silence they used to have at the foot of Hogan's Bend. It reduced barge costs on the Alabama River by however many trips are made over that ten-mile stretch every year, and it will continue to save costs so long as there is river traffic.

The price of this silence and these savings was that it cost the system sixty acres of bottomland hardwood and nailed the hides of two fishing camp operators to the barn door.

The island made the world safer for pelicans but more restrictive for oysters, and I am really not qualified to decide which is the most valuable. I must admit I have both an opinion and a preference, however, because I never ate a pelican.

Everything has a cost. Somebody has to pay it, but the way it often seems to work out is that the one who calls the tune is not always the one who pays the piper.

Like Donne said, "No man is an island, entire of itself."

13

The Colonel's Daughter

O NE OF THE THINGS that is difficult for any man to realize is the fact that by and large, other people
have very little interest in either his business or his
actions.

Paranoids disagree. They feel that not only is
everybody watching but that most of them are engaged in con-
spiracies. New fathers disagree because they think every living
person wants to look at pictures of their children. New grandpar-
ents disagree in a league all by themselves because they restrict
their conversation to the antics of their heirs and assigns in the
generation that is once removed.

Except to your doctor, your stockbroker, and those persons
who are slated for a share of the estate, the details of your health
are not exactly items of absorbing interest unless you happen to
be a public figure, and Bum Phillips hit it right on the head
when he pointed out that attendance at your funeral is going to
depend very largely upon the weather.

To be perfectly blunt about it, you and I and everyone else
we know all operate mostly as faces in the crowd. Nobody really
gives a damn what we do, say, or feel, with the exception of
members of our immediate family— and usually not every one of
them. This may hurt your feelings and hurt them badly, but unfortunately, the cookie crumbles in just such a fashion.

Those of us with offspring, however, find the thought
processes and actions of those offspring to be not only ab-

sorbingly interesting and of premier importance, but almost wholly without fault of any kind.

All of which goes a long way toward explaining why most of the troubles experienced by the members of hunting clubs can be traced to a single fact: the conduct of the sons of the members.

This conduct, more than anything else, is the factor most responsible for moving the dislike index between certain club members over into the hatred zone. It does so because only the father can find extenuating circumstances to excuse the actions of the son.

Everybody loves the ten-year-old son of a club member. Ten-year-old boys are friendly, willing, obliging, take up little room, and, as a general rule, hunt only in the company of the father who considers himself responsible for the boy's actions.

People tend to pontificate over the posthunt bourbon about how pleasant it is to have the little fellows sitting literally at our feet, soaking up the crumbs of wisdom that fall gently on the hearth stone, and speaking only when spoken to. Always available to poke up the fire and freshen up the glasses, preparing themselves to take our places in the long brown line when we have all gone to that great hunting ground in the sky. Years and years from now, of course.

These golden moments at the fireside generally last until the ten-year-olds get to be eighteen or so, go off to college, and come back for the weekend, bringing fraternity brothers with them to join us in the hunt.

All of a sudden at that point, what used to be a friendly, obliging, tousled little tyke becomes a gawky, callow, opinionated pain in the ass.

People begin to remember W. C. Fields's deathless line, "Any man who hates dogs and children can't be all bad."

They even recall the one-word crusher used when he was asked how he liked children and he answered, "Boiled."

Even softhearted candy asses like me, remembering myself at the age of seventeen being roughed up by professionals in the armed forces of the United States, have thought how nice it would be to keep a small, well-bred war going on somewhere all the time so we could have a place to send these clods to get their rough edges knocked off.

They seem to show us their worst side during the Christmas vacation. Most colleges give three weeks or so off during that time, most all the hunting seasons in our end of the world are open, and camp houses fill up with loudmouthed barbarians who are rude to the help, eat up all the groceries, sign in for all the choice places, overstay their welcome, bend the club rules in all sorts of devious ways, and, in general, encourage a man to turn to Buddhism because Buddhists have no Christmas vacation to bother about.

Every bit of this is conducted under the benevolent jurisdiction of the member who happens to be the father of the clod who brought this plague of locusts down upon us in the first place. Not a single bit of it is offensive to him, because the perfection inherent in his own children serves to mask the tiny flaws that may possibly occur in any of their friends.

If you are fortunate enough to have all of your offspring born as girl children, then virtually none of this becomes a load you will ever have to carry.

There is only one tiny disadvantage with girls and that is when the child accompanies you on hunts, and you are a member of a small club with an even smaller clubhouse, there is a little bit of difficulty with bathroom arrangements.

Get past that minor flaw, and it is "strew on her roses, roses, and never a spray of yew," just like Matthew Arnold wrote a hundred and forty years ago.

In the early years, until they get to be about twelve, as the father of daughters you have infinitely the better of the two sexes. Your interest at this stage is in companionship rather than physical strength.

But Kipling was precisely correct when he pointed out that the female of the species is more deadly than the male.

Little girls have not yet reached the age when they feel compelled to put the veneer of ladylike reticence over their innate bloody-mindedness.

They will rap crippled ducks in the head, wring the necks of wounded doves, or prowl around the insides of turkeys during the gut extraction stage with the same relaxed and ladylike aplomb with which they will pour champagne at bridesmaid's luncheons ten years later.

They are absolutely as quick, precisely as agile, just as perfectly prepared to do the dirty work, and far more cold-blooded than little boys usually are at that age. The only thing they don't do as well is the heavy lifting and that, after all, is why you have gone along in the first place.

And then, after they have gotten past the unisex age and have definitely turned into girls, you are never going to be asked to inflict half the population of the Kappa house upon the hunting club during the Christmas holidays.

A lot of the girl children at that age will start to develop different habits. They begin to specialize in afternoon dove shoots and are willing to take up the practice of following bird dogs only after the sun has come out and melted the frost.

Some of them, at this stage, have completely lost their taste for watching the world wake up from inside a duck blind or being in the woods thirty minutes before the first cardinal whistles during the first week in April. But whatever it is they hunt at this age, they hunt singly. They do not come in bunches, like bananas, principally because there are not enough of them still interested to form a crowd. And even the ones who have temporarily retired from active participation in the hunt remember the ground rules, are aware of the tactics, and can carry on intelligent, posthunt conversations.

Unless they are cold-bloodedly sticking the knife in on purpose, they think right. After being told how many turkeys you heard gobble, they never make comments like, "Well, if you heard that many, why didn't you shoot some of them?"

Even if they never come back to hunting, and some don't, you are light years ahead.

You had them during the early good years, and even if these happen to be followed by nothing, there are no bad memories to rub the gloss off the early shine.

We had the boat before we had the girl, and at the beginning of her career, the Colonel's daughter spent a lot of her early days involved in river operations with small boats. A boat, in point of fact, was the first powered vehicle she was allowed to operate alone, even with someone else in the vehicle to take the blame.

In a splendid example of how the bend in the sapling creates the form of the resulting tree, she exhibited the same reckless disregard for life, limb, and property with the boat that she was to exhibit while running a golf cart two years later.

My wife said that during the conduct of boat-handling lessons, you could hear me yelling at her from Boat House Landing to the mouth of Pine Log Creek, a distance of nearly a mile.

The answer, of course, was that I only yelled at people who deserved it, and with a daughter like we had, I could only thank God that I had been lucky enough to spend as many years as I had on a parade ground, giving instructions to an entire battalion over the sound of the band, to help me develop the proper volume.

God put certain daughters on this earth whose temperament is such that nothing weaker than a parade ground bellow can adequately catch their attention. The volume of my voice just happens to serve as a remarkable example of the actions of an all-wise providence, who came up with the solution some years before the arrival of the problem.

She was in the boat the morning when bream were on the bed in Clearwater Lake and we went through fifty crickets in fifty-four minutes by the clock.

She fished. I paddled, took off fish, baited the hook with fresh crickets, and passed the cold drinks in my spare time.

Things moved so fast that I lost any opportunity to close the lid on the ice chest. After the first eight or ten fish were in the box, I just left the lid open. By the time we got to twenty-five, if a fish was not bigger than one we already had in the box, I simply dropped him back in the water and rebaited.

Normally, when it comes to fishing, the height of her boredom threshold can be measured with a micrometer. This day was an example of the kind that would have measured it in yards, if there had been time enough to stop and measure.

The Colonel's daughter and all the rest of the family—Père, Mère, and Fido—were on the way to the boat that memorable February afternoon when our springer flushed the two turkeys.

The boat had been left on the shore of the unnamed lake at the end of what was called the Rogers' Mill Road—whoever the hell Rogers was and whatever the hell kind of mill he had—at the end of the duck season. It had been there for nearly a month and a half when one afternoon, just prowling around, I went by the boat and saw that the beavers had done a pretty successful job of eating the corners off it.

I have had shabby treatment of this sort from beavers before and since.

As light as juniper boards are, it is perfectly possible to carry a couple of three by eights, eight feet long, in the back of a pickup to help you over mud holes. They are light enough to manhandle over a bad place in the road, if it is short, and while they are too fragile to serve as bridges, they serve admirably as runners.

I have, on occasion, left one at a blown-out culvert, or at a place where one end of a bridge has been undermined so you could use it as a foot log for a short distance. In all of these cases, the piece of timber, if left in place for several weeks, gets gnawed by beavers—sometimes severely.

There cannot possibly be any sustenance in bone-dry ten-year-old juniper. There is no sap, and I cannot make myself believe beavers lie awake at night thinking up fresh troubles to create for hunters and come up with the scheme of gnawing up their boats and bridge runners.

I don't like beavers. I rank them in the same category with social diseases and cottonmouth moccasins, but I have never specifically hunted up a beaver and made these thoughts known to him. Why they would gather across a section and a half of timber to help eat my boat, I have no idea, but they did.

They gnawed both upper corners at the transom, a substantial part of the rail outside the gunwales, a chunk out of the prow right up at the top, and an area as big as both your hands—halfway between the bottom and the gunwale—that came within a quarter inch of going all the way through one of the side boards.

Nothing that could not be repaired with a lavish use of epoxy, sanded and covered with paint, but a signal example of the same kind of pointless vandalism that causes bears to destroy mountain cabins.

The four of us drove up to the woods one Sunday afternoon, parked, and walked in. In the last two hundred yards before we got to where the boat was pulled up on the shore, the springer puppy ran up two turkey gobblers who let him get his nose almost between them before they flew.

For a dog only three months old, whose previous experience had been limited to slate-colored juncos and chipping sparrows in the backyard, it was a substantial upgrade. It scared the living hell out of him.

There is something about turkeys that makes a person's first exposure to them at close range a memorable event. Memorable to the extent that he wants to keep reliving the incident in his mind and causes him, moreover, to tell you the story again and again until you want to shriek, "For Christ's sake! You told me already!"

Evidently, they have the same effect on dogs.

After the initial terrified recoil from the flush, he pranced down the ridge in the direction they had gone, barking hysterically for the first two hundred yards or so, and then came back and told us all about it. In barks, naturally.

For the next hour or so, while I mended the gnawed places and both the distaff elements sat on a log and gave instructions, he would reenact the flush, run barking down the ridge to rescatter the already-vanished turkeys, and then come back and tell us about it all over again.

He reminded you of nothing so much as a hunter who improves his story continuously as time passes. His behavior grew steadily more forceful, and there at the end he was acting as if he had taken the scent the minute we got out of the car and had run a quarter of a mile at a dead gallop to effect the flush.

Any story, told either by man or dog, is almost bound to improve with age so long as a strict adherence to the truth is not held to be obligatory.

The Colonel's daughter was in the boat the September morning we got lost in a shut-down fog trying to get into Bay Minette Basin for the opening day of teal season. A fog thick enough to let you tell up from down only by watching which way the boat paddle went when you held it out in front of you and let go.

She was in the boat the morning I set the all-time world's record for the single-scull, juniper duckboat, two-hundred-yard dash, crewed by father and daughter, open class.

Before the old clubhouse burned down, there was a blackboard on the front porch. It was expected that those hunting anything—but turkeys in particular—would sign into the woods on the board, describe the area they intended to hunt, stay in that location, and sign out by erasing their names from the board when they left.

Such conventions on turkeys are rigidly respected. No one can tell until you come out and say so whether or not you are working with a turkey, and no one needs to have someone drive up and engage in friendly conversation when the drive up runs off a turkey you have been working for an hour and a half.

If a person took a guest who was hunting in a different place, it was expected that that area would be mentioned as well. Two people hunting together would simply sign in as Jones and guest, or whatever. When the Colonel's daughter and I went together, we always signed the board as Kelly & Kelly.

Coming out, if we had been unsuccessful, after she had erased the names she always wrote, "Turkeys 26, Hunters 0," on the bottom of the sign-out board. When we won, she signed out as "Hunters 1, Turkeys 0." Once, and only once, I considered we had tied.

Kelly & Kelly had signed the board and crossed the river at Pierce's Landing on Easter Saturday morning because I had heard a turkey gobble once after he flew up to roost the evening before on that side of the river.

We crossed in the dark, tied up to the west bank, and heard the turkey gobble twenty minutes after daylight. Just as we got to him (he had been close when we first heard him) it thundered in the northwest.

Cold fronts here all come from the northwest and are usually preceded by two or three days of south or southeast winds. Fast-moving cold fronts are frequently accompanied by severe thunderstorms and pronounced line squalls, and the temperature can sometimes drop thirty degrees in thirty minutes.

Leaving out the possibility of lightning strikes, you never want to get wet in the rain and then rattle your teeth out shaking in the cold wind after it shifts, so I unilaterally called off the turkey hunt, and we started back to the boat.

Called it off without eliciting a smidgen of back talk, as a matter of fact, because the light was no longer increasing, but was dimming, the sky was beginning to take on a distinctly eerie look, we began to hear the wind and rain coming from the northwest, and it felt just like a dandy time to go back to the cave.

We got to the boat in a fast trot, got in, and shoved off, and I had taken maybe three strokes with the paddle when the wind shifted 180 degrees almost instantly, switched into the northwest, and within twenty seconds was blowing in thirty-knot gusts.

When we got fifty yards out into the river, we could see the black line of the squall coming over our shoulders and hear the wind in the trees behind us. There were single leaves and small twigs with two or three leaves attached to them blowing all the way across the river.

Paddling into the teeth of that wind would have been impossible, but luckily it wasn't necessary. It was pushing us in the direction we intended to go, and although I am relying on my own memory, I really believe that at one time I had the boat up on the step. With enough wind to help, you really can paddle one fast enough to make it plane.

Whatever time you happen to believe is the absolute minimum required for paddling a juniper duckboat two hundred yards is way too high. Believe me, we lowered it, although the record, being wind assisted, cannot be considered official.

We didn't even get wet.

The rain was far enough behind the wind to let us get the boat tied off and run to the car before the heavens opened.

There are things that happen to you in life that stick in your memory. Odd incidents, some triumphs, some sadnesses. Often a single glimpse of something sticks the best of all.

In her younger days, she had the guts of a burglar and was fearless. Sometimes fearless beyond the bounds of reasonable intelligence.

But the incident had been truly scary—that kind of weather tends to be—and driving out in the car she had a distinctly contemplative look on her face. She turned to me and said: "Daddy, did it scare you?"

And I answered, "I was okay until that old lady in the long black dress, riding the bicycle with the little dog in the basket blew by. I got to admit that right then I did begin to worry a little."

The way her face changed at the remark, the way the pinched look of concern was replaced by the sunniest of smiles, constitutes one of those things that will stick in my memory all the rest of the way to the boneyard.

Any time I want to see that grin, any time I want to resavor that particular moment, all I have to do is close my eyes.

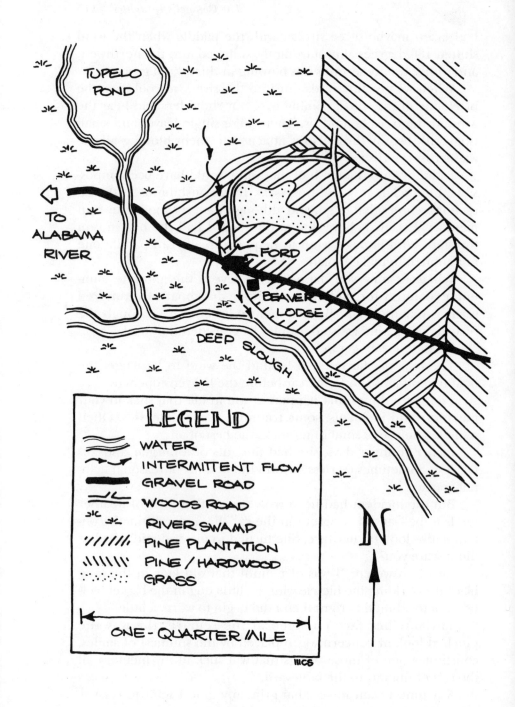

TUPELO POND

TO ALABAMA RIVER

FORD

BEAVER LODGE

DEEP SLOUGH

LEGEND

〰〰 WATER
➴ INTERMITTENT FLOW
▬▬ GRAVEL ROAD
〰 WOODS ROAD
⋉⋉ RIVER SWAMP
/////// PINE PLANTATION
\\\\\\\ PINE / HARDWOOD
⋅⋅⋅⋅⋅⋅ GRASS

ONE - QUARTER MILE

N

14

Without a Boat at All

ONE OF THE MORE curious situations that arises when you address the matter of the measurement of area is the complete lack of appreciation most people have concerning the size of an acre. People talk about acres all the time. Land is bought, sold, and taxed by the acre. Various phrases using the word have even crept into the vernacular, things like "Hell's half acre," for example. But when someone tries to describe exactly what an acre looks like or come up with a recognizable simile to help describe its size, it becomes clear that there is a vast body of ignorance.

An acre is a football field, less the end zones, with one end cut off at the nine-yard line. To put it in better perspective, if your shotgun has an effective range of forty yards and you sit down in the woods and lean your back up against a tree, the half circle in gunshot in front of you covers half an acre.

A single acre in the middle of the desert or as a part of the grass prairies of the Midwest is a nonentity. Fill an acre with trees or with briar patches, however, or pack it with granite rocks that must be reduced to gravel to let a road go through, and it becomes a very large area indeed.

Some acres, in addition to being large, seem to resemble certain people. They don't just lie there or stand around and constitute faces in the crowd. Something unusual always seems to be happening where they are.

I happen to be acquainted with an acre that, while maybe

117

not holding the world's championship for weird, clearly qualifies in the top rank of unusual and has been doing so for the past twenty years. It first called itself to my attention when it gave me the opportunity to match a memorable, smart-ass remark.

Some years ago, the State of Alabama, in an attempt to get a better handle on the causes of forest fires, devised a form and required each forest ranger or patrolman to complete the form, on the spot, immediately after a forest fire had been suppressed. One of the questions to be answered called for an opinion as to the cause of the fire.

Such a determination is outrageously difficult to make, to say the least. There are some causes that are immediately evident—those fires caused by lightning for instance, or when someone has been burning off a field and the fire jumps the plowed line he put inside the fences. The sparks from coal-burning trains made it easy, back when trains burned coal and assuming someone was there to watch the fire start. But by and large, the origins of forest fires are cloudy at best, and the cause-of-fire blank to be filled on the form was filled largely by guesses, only some of which could be called educated.

The heat began to be applied from above, as it always is, by some of those persons always present in a higher headquarters who specialize in demanding specifically detailed intelligence that is nearly impossible to gather.

A forest patrolman of my acquaintance, happily possessed of a blithe disregard of constituted authority, and with a whimsical sense of humor and a turn of phrase to match, filled in such a blank on such a form with a world-class remark.

Very neatly printed, in the space calling for cause of fire, he wrote: "Chicken pecked a match. Think it was a rooster."

I would love to have been the man who thought of that and was then, and still am, consumed with envy of an intellect that can come up with a zapper of such pungency.

Some years later, not precisely in imitation of his remark but clearly inspired by its example, I had almost the same opportunity, and it was afforded by the unusual acre we were just talking about.

The acre lies just at the break in terrain where a woods road leaves the mixed pine-hardwood uplands and drops down into the river swamp. The change in altitude is no more than five feet, but so far as species composition and ground conditions are concerned, it could very well be a hundred.

Crossing the road there, at the very edge of the timber-type change, is a slough, forded by the road, that can change from being a graveled dip in the road at low river stages to a running stream chest-deep in the middle at high ones.

There is a forty-acre pine plantation there, in the very last of the mixed pine-hardwood type. In cases of extremely high rivers, the last two or three acres in the bottom corner of this plantation are sometimes knee-deep in flood water and stay that way for a week or ten days. Pine can't take any degree of flooding to speak of, which is why you find none in the river swamp, but it can take it for a week or so, so long as the flooded weeks do not come too close together.

Twenty years ago, just after this plantation had been established, I came out of the woods on the upper end of the field at a point being some several feet in elevation above the lower end. The river was in flood, and way down there in the flooded bottom corner, I saw a mullet jumping over the freshly planted pine seedlings.

Mullet jump over pine trees only upon the rarest of occasions, principally due to the fact that the normal habitats of the two species seldom coincide. Because the maximum ordinate of the trajectory of a jumping mullet is about three feet, such a co-incidence must necessarily occur while the pine trees are very small.

When I was a boy on this coast, mullet were caught in cast nets, and it was held as an article of faith that they could not be caught on hook and line. What we dullards on the coast did not know was that mullet migrate upstream into fresh water—they are commonly seen forty to fifty miles above salt water—and that they were, and are, being caught along sandbars in the river by the dozens on hook and line. The bait used is a small piece of a worm, the hook is about the size of that used for bream, and they are caught in about eighteen inches of water. It makes a man wonder how many articles now firmly held in faith along the coast are just as wrong as the no-mullet-on-a-hook-and-line hypothesis was in 1940.

A saltwater mullet will jump from the water repeatedly, sometimes with four or five jumps occurring in succession. I have no idea why they do this, but then, considering the gaps in my knowledge concerning mullet behavior in general, this last should not come as a surprise.

Upriver mullet jump as much as saltwater mullet, and the mullet I saw, aloft over the pine trees, jumped over several because he was moving along a row of planted trees at the time of the observation.

When trees are planted in plantations, there is a survival survey done at the end of the second year, and sometimes one is made at the end of the third. The purpose of these surveys is to ascertain the number of trees that have survived the first couple of seasons and to decide whether a replanting program will be necessary. In conducting the survey, a number of one-hundredth acre plots are taken; the number of live and dead trees in each plot is tallied; and if live trees have been damaged, a notation is made as to what, in the cruiser's opinion, caused the damage.

I was therefore able to put a survival plot in this plantation, in the area where I had seen the jumping fish, with a notation that became a part of the official records and was carried as such for nearly twenty years. The notation said, "Plot number 14, seedling no. 6 damaged. Terminal shoot broken off. Think it was a mullet."

After trees are planted and the survival studies made, there is no real reason for anyone to visit the site for several years, let alone look at the records. Roads and fire lines will be maintained, and in the event of a wildfire, another survival survey will be made to see what is left. But the crop is effectively laid by until the time comes for control burns or until the cruises are made to see if volumes have grown to the point that thinnings may be possible. The pleasure, therefore, that I was able to derive from the knowledge that the damage statement rested in the records was private in nature, but was no less enjoyable because of that.

Some ten years after the mullet incident, the acre called attention to itself again when it became the site of the only dryland beaver house I have ever seen.

Beavers usually build their houses of sticks and limbs, held together by mud and beaver spit, well out in the pond behind the dam. The entrance to the house is made under water to deny entrance to predators. Most beaver predators, being either canine or feline, cannot swim under water with any degree of competence. The beavers on the magic acre built their house on dry land, six feet back from the edge of the slough.

The entrance tunnel came from the slough, and they didn't bother to put the entrance hole under water. The entrance began as an open ditch, and you could walk to the edge of the slough and see the ditch come out of the water and turn into a tunnel just before it ended. It was perfectly possible to walk up to the house and rap on top of it with a stick. This invariably caused rustling and moving-about sounds from inside the house, all clearly audible, and sometimes there would even be whining and other vocalizing noises coming from inside as well.

Not only did they make no attempt to hide the entrance— even normal beavers never hide the house but leave it sticking up out of the water like a low, untidy haystack—they made no attempt to be secretive about their presence.

The plantation was thinned at the age of eighteen, taking out every third row and some of the inferior trees in the rows being left. The beavers existed in perfect harmony with the logging operation, although I had no reports of them sitting out on the front porch in the sunshine in rocking chairs to watch. After thinnings, plantations are generally more subject to lose trees because of wind throw than they were before, and two years after this area was thinned we had a major hurricane. So much of the remaining timber was blown down that it was decided to cut what was left and start over. There was the usual amount of understory that had developed under the old plantation, and during normal site preparation activities, the dry-land beaver house was disked up and turned under.

Again, there were no reports of infuriated beavers attacking the site preparation machinery, but I would not have been the least bit surprised to hear of it. The way this colony had acted all their lives, it was obvious they felt they were the owners and had allowed the rest of us to be in the woods from time to time only on sufferance and because of their innate good nature. It is my considered judgment that the only reason they moved at all was because they felt that when the hurricane blew down all the trees, it ruined the neighborhood.

A sensible beaver family would simply move downstream,

build another dam, put a house in the middle of the resulting pond, and press on from there. I would not make book on anything that simple with this set of deviants. They are bound to go and build a dam somewhere that floods a boat-launching ramp or an equipment shed or the approaches to a new bridge on the highway. We have not heard the last from them and, as soon as the newly planted trees are ten feet tall, I am convinced some of their descendants will be back on the magic acre, this time probably trying to put their house in the middle of the gravel road.

You should not get the impression that the magic acre lay dormant from the time of the airborne mullet to the incident of the dry-land beavers; it is far too busy for that. Just after the gravel road crosses the dip—the crossing that can vary from being a low place in the road to a waist-deep stream and occupy any stage in between—there is a place south of the gravel road, on the river side of the ford, that holds a turkey or two every spring, every year. It is a splendid place for turkeys to roost, and the terrain, like a strategically located fairway trap on a good golf course, is located in the precise place and with the exact configuration designed to cause the maximum amount of trouble.

It is a trapezoid of about ten acres in size with a half-dozen spruce pines along the south side of the road that serve as excellent roost trees. A turkey roosting in any of these trees has a perfect view up and down the road. The road itself offers an attractive landing ground as he pitches down, and, because there is a screen of low trees along the side of the trapezoid formed by the intermittent slough, you are tempted to wade the slough when the water is only knee-deep to be sure you can see what goes on down in the lower corner.

Three times out of four it is a mistake, because three nights out of four something is roosting in one of the trees along the road and sits up there, absorbed with interest, watching you wade over.

If you elect not to wade across and accept the blind area behind the screen of trees along the slough to your left, a turkey will pitch down in there and gobble for thirty minutes and never come into the road in front of you to let you see him.

If you go early enough to cross the water in the black dark and get set up without running something off the roost along the side of the road, turkeys can pitch down north of the road, fly across the slough to the north of you, and then go stand in the grass patch in the middle of the plantation and gobble until they break your heart.

One of the solutions—the kind of situation that caused me to get a boat and leave it in the swamp in the first place—is the fact that you can cross the slough by boat, two hundred yards before you get to the ford in the road, and thereby gain access to the blind area in the southeast corner of the trapezoid without showing either your hand or your face in the road at the crossing. This can work, unless the river is high enough to make the current in the slough too swift to paddle across.

It is a remarkable example of a combination of terrain, visibility, and a surface appearance of offered opportunity that treacherously manages to catch you on the wrong foot and keeps you off balance most of the time.

There are rare exceptions, and last year was one of them.

The dip in the road was nearly at full depth and in full flood. There was still dry land available in the area across the water. The afternoon before, I had sat in the road at the lower end of the plantation until full dark, had heard two turkeys fly up to roost in the extreme southwest corner of the trapezoid, and knew there were none roosting in the trees along the side of the road.

I was there the next morning before daylight. I changed from boots to chest-high waders in the middle of the road, in the dark, two hundred yards before I got to the crossing.

In the middle of the crossing, with the water waist-deep and things as dark as they are in a coal mine, I realized the water was a good deal deeper than it looked and the current was a knot or so faster than it normally ran. In the middle of the flow, it became necessary to half turn to face the current and lean forward and shuffle sideways in order to be able to stay in the road. It was another of those prime examples of how some of us have simply grown older, the additional years not having been accompanied by additional wisdom. It brought back to mind one of my father's infuriating but accurate statements to the effect that the older I got, the worse I got.

The decision not to try to cross in the boat had been correct. The flow of the current was such that it would have jammed you into the trees on the south side of the road before you could effect the crossing.

Current running at the speed it was that morning will sometimes set up eddies and carve out holes in the middle of the road three feet deeper than the rest of the roadbed. Stepping into one of these unexpectedly, in the dark, wearing chest-high waders and carrying a shotgun, would be at the very least an exhilarating experience. You might even get a chance to drink a little more water than you felt you could comfortably handle.

Being dumb but lucky one more time, I got across and moved just far enough south to get out of the road, still be able to see down it, and have a view of the area across the slough I had just crossed. I didn't take the waders off, not wanting to spend the time or make the noise struggling out of anything.

Just at daylight, a turkey gobbled south of me exactly one time. It sounded as if you had dropped a gobbling box down a flight of no more than three steps. The last of the three notes was half choked off, and you couldn't have heard it at a quarter of a mile to save your life. I tree-yelped in return, and there was a very little yelping in answer. About fifteen minutes later, there were a couple of muted clucks.

He came into view at about two hundred yards, and it must have taken him thirty minutes to come from two hundred yards to forty. He would take a couple of tiny steps, drop both wings and strut, turn completely around, look in all directions, and take two more six-inch steps. The rate of march was almost at the speed of a mile a week. Simply looking at it was nerve-wracking. Because he made no other sound, if he had not been in sight all the time, you would have been sorely tempted to give up and go try somewhere else.

I pulled the trigger at a quarter past seven. He was four years old and had extremely sharp spurs that were beginning to curve up sharply. There were no worn primaries to show he had been strutting and dragging his wings very extensively. His craw had a noticeable amount of green sprouts and old acorns, showing he was still eating regularly. He was either somewhat past the age of chasing girls or else he was slow to begin.

Coming back across the slough was much easier than going in. I couldn't see the bottom in the middle of the ford then either, but things always appear less foreboding in the bright sunshine. I have a length of parachute cord tied to a hardwood stick to help carry turkeys. Both his feet go in the loop in the end of the cord, and the stick gives you something to hold on to while he is hanging over your shoulder. In the middle of the ford he got very light all of a sudden, and I realized that big turkeys, hung over one shoulder, float in water that is waist deep. You depend on water to float a string of ducks, but I had never floated a turkey before. The principle is identical, it is just that the experience is so unexpected.

Coming to the last few steps of the ford, out of the main current and with the turkey again beginning to make his weight felt on my back, something small flew across the ford from behind me and landed in the edge of the grass patch on the other side. I really didn't pay it much attention until it was joined by several more.

They were snipe.

By the time I had gotten back to where I had left the boots and changed to waders and had put the turkey down, I had seen a dozen. I sat at the side of the road and watched at least two or three dozen snipe fly back and forth, landing in the edge of the grass patch just out of the water, trading back and forth across the new plantation like the midafternoon arrivals in a very good dove field.

There was nice firm ground underfoot, there was no ankle-deep mud to struggle with, there was a comfortable place to sit, and there was the equivalent of clipped lawn for them to fall on after you shot them. I have never been on a comfortable snipe hunt in my life, but if there has ever been an opportunity, that morning must have come as close as it can get.

Obviously, on March 31st in this latitude, snipe are on their way back north. Our snipe season closes the last day of February, and there is no doubt but that the elimination of spring shooting has had a major effect on the restoration of our waterfowl. The Congress of the United States has made no provision that permits a citizen to reopen a spring migratory bird season on his own authority, because of unusual circumstances.

I am aware that several major religions have, as a matter of iron-clad dogma, the tenet that no man is allowed to be tempted beyond the ability of flesh and blood to withstand. But of all the game birds in North America, these two species stand at the absolute outer limits of the bell curve, at both ends.

A three-ounce snipe and an eighteen-pound turkey shot on the same day within a half hour of one another on an acre of land where mullet jump over pine trees would make a tale a man could add to his repertoire and tell as one of his better after-dinner stories the rest of the way to the boneyard.

As badly as I wanted to do it, I did not shoot a snipe. Not because I consider myself to be a responsible, law-abiding citizen. Nor because I believe that a single snipe, shot slightly after normal shooting hours, could have all that much effect on the brood stock, even though thirty-one days after normal shooting hours might be considered somewhat longer than slightly.

The single thing that kept me honest was the matter of equipment.

I shoot turkeys with a three-inch twelve-gauge and two ounces of number four shot. It would be as inappropriate to shoot snipe with four drams of powder and two ounces of fours as it would be to smash wild violets with a ten-pound sledgehammer or shoot green-wing teal with an eight-inch howitzer. So I restricted myself to unloading the gun, swinging on several left to rights, and clicking the trigger on an empty chamber.

But if I had had in my pocket, last All Fool's Eve, a single three-dram cartridge loaded with an ounce of eights, I would most surely have done something I could not talk about in public.

And there would have to be entered in the books a modification to the existing rules of the limits of temptation that normal flesh and blood can be expected to withstand.

Furthermore, some of my after-dinner conversations, at least those conducted in the company of close friends, might now be following a different direction altogether.

15

The Key of H

AWAY BACK IN THE DIM and distant past, in an era so long ago that it could legitimately be described as once upon a time, I was young enough to be sung to sleep by my father.

His repertoire was comprised wholly of tearjerkers sung in a tempo that matched the movement of the rocking chair and had to be heard to be believed. For instance:

In "The Baggage Coach Ahead," the father tells the complaining passenger that he cannot get the child's mother to stop it from crying, because the mother is in her coffin up in the baggage coach.

"Scalded to Death by Steam" meant exactly what it said. The engineer of old No. 97 was found beneath the wreck with his hand on the throttle in precisely that condition.

"Break the News to Mother" was the last letter of a young soldier, wounded and dying in the hospital, telling his mother to snuff out the candle in the window because he wouldn't be coming home at all.

Nobody had a bit of fun in any of these epics, or in any of his other selections. Taken literally, they could mark a child for life, give him a case of the glooms that would last all the way to voting age. I can only suppose that the 1920s considered them calming to the lively infant.

In addition to the fact that Daddy's material was inferior,

there was the matter of the quality of his voice. Unfortunately, that was not exactly top of the line either.

A vacuum cleaner on ground balls, a genius with a kite in light airs, and a consummate artist with a cast net not withstanding, put a song on his tongue and a child in his lap and you were leaning on a frail reed indeed.

He didn't know this. He said people objected to his singing because they couldn't understand him. It was a mile over their heads. He said it was because he sang in the key of H.

The key of H is composed of sounds completely outside the normal probabilities curve and is almost unknown to those conventional, stuffy, music teachers who insist on stopping things at G. Nor is the key of H restricted to music alone. There are all sorts of improbable things out there. Things like Rogers Hornsby hitting over .400 three times in five years or Bobby Jones winning both opens and both amateurs in 1930.

My own singing, according to the Colonel's daughter, was at least the equal of her grandfather's. Although I specialized in "Lili Marlene," stolen from the German army, and "Flow Gently Sweet Afton," stolen from Robert Burns—thereby sparing her the trauma of nineteenth-century tragedies, preserving her id from irreparable harm, and putting her to sleep quickly—she has never appreciated it. In fact, I have heard her say it was necessary to go to sleep quickly. It was the only way to get away from the music.

Evidently, singing in the key of H is an inheritable trait.

So is an appreciation of some of the other examples of H. Mysterious happenings, anomalies, things beyond the curve, things like the incident of the pasture ducks.

Two of us had parked the pickup in the northeast corner of a hundred-acre pasture one December afternoon and had separated to cover the ridges that led away from there to try to scatter a drove of turkeys for the next morning. I found enough scratching to qualify as site preparation, some hillsides looking as if they had been raked and piled, but nothing specific. So, at fifteen minutes before flying-up time, I decided to go and listen from the point of an extremely long ridge that ran north and overlooked a hardwood flat of nearly four hundred acres.

On the very point of the ridge there was a three-acre stand of sawlog-sized shortleaf, and everybody arrived there at the same time. Me, on the little trail coming up from the south and an outstanding drove of turkeys coming out of the hollow on the left-hand side.

Everybody who came to the meeting was surprised.

As they began to flush off the end of the ridge, I shot, twice, and they fanned out over the hollow in front of me in almost a perfect semicircle.

If there was one turkey, there were fifty.

I stood there, after the explosion, and mentally went around the semicircle to reconstruct how many had flown between such-and-such a tree and its neighboring snag, how many between the sun and a particularly bushy-topped shortleaf, and so on. Every way I added it up I came back to fifty, and I couldn't recall any group of more than two or three at any point on the half circle, which meant I didn't even have to go down into either hollow to complete the scattering. I had done it all at once, with two shots.

One of the most pleasant occupations known to man is the process of concocting a scheme to brag on yourself, using the clipped understatement and the throw-away line, after you have done something truly outstanding. I had my story well in hand at just about the time I got back to the pasture fence, a quarter of a mile west of where we had parked the truck. It was still pretty light out in the open, and just as I stepped across the fence, a little flock of wood ducks crossed the pasture south of me and flew over the corner at the truck, ten yards high.

In the five minutes it took me to walk over there, three more little groups had crossed the pasture and flown out at the corner, the last of the three having to gain some altitude to get over the fence posts.

Jim was standing at the corner with a strange look on his face, and as I walked up he said, "Those ducks are landing on the ground out there on the point of this ridge."

As soon as I expressed firm disbelief, he said it again.

I was in the middle of a complaint about people who start drinking before the hunt is over, get tiddly and tell outrageous stories about fictitious natural phenomena to their friends, who know better, when I was interrupted.

Four wood ducks came over us at a height you could have reached with the gun barrel, cupped their wings as they passed, and pitched down on the ridge sixty yards away. We heard them thump when they landed.

There is a minor timber type common all across the upper coastal plain. It is generally small, less than five acres in size, and is usually an outcropping of Eustis Sands. It is called a Water Oak ridge.

Eustis Sand is a coarse sand, pretty low in fertility, and generally dry enough to grow a little prickly pear cactus. The density of the oak and the infertility of the soil restrict the understory, and except for the cactus, it will usually be perfectly clean under the trees. Because the site is so sterile, the trees peak out at about eighteen inches in diameter.

The ridge next to us was one of these. There had been a heavy red oak acorn crop that year, and you couldn't walk without crushing four or five water oak acorns with each step. The point of the ridge was covered with ducks. You could hear them chuckling to one another as they fed. There were so many you could hear them walking in the leaves.

I know some ducks feed at night, but I never knew that wood ducks prowled around among the cactus and ate water oak acorns off dry ridges in the black dark.

We talked about going out to the end of the ridge and running them off, but it was way too dark by then to tell which way they would go, so we walked away and left them at dinner.

It opens up whole paragraphs of unknowns.

Do they do this often? Do they spend the night on the ground? If they leave, how do they see well enough to land in the regular roosts in the dark? With all day to do it in, why do they wait until dark and feed on-top of a ridge within half a mile of their normal roost pond?

It is well out from under the probabilities curve. It is a prime example of one of those things in the key of H. But there is a better example, and that is the one of the invisible turkey.

There used to be a fairly widespread school of thought—I have even seen it in print—that game birds possessed the capacity to withhold their scent. I have never believed it—considered it preposterous and lumped it in with hoop snakes.

Nor do I believe that turkeys can burrow underground, like moles, or render themselves invisible; although over the years, in fits of frustration, I have accused them of both.

But there have been moments.

Last spring I had a turkey I had gone to every day for a week. He gobbled regularly and often, every morning in the same place, just across a slough that the boat let me cross in a half-dozen strokes of the paddle and right on the edge of a mixed pine and hardwood stand that reached down to the backwater.

Every morning he would be the first turkey to gobble. Just about the time I would get to him and sit down, another turkey would begin to gobble away to the north, always on my side of the slough, but always late.

There is a tactical rule that says you ought not to leave one to go to another, unless the one you sat down to gives you some reason to suspect he may be hopeless. Gobbling fifty times on the roost and a hundred on the ground certainly gives you no such indication. Two or three mornings I was severely tempted, but never to the extent to cause me to be fickle.

Leaping up to go to every other gobble you hear, while giving you the opportunity to view all kinds of new scenery and limbering up your running muscles, is exceptionally restful to the muscles in your thumb and forefinger—the ones you pick turkey feathers with.

Then one morning Old Faithful stood mute, and the turkey to the north was the first one to gobble. I have another rule. I always go to the first turkey. Always. Not only is it better to take sure cash before probable credit, it is also considered good manners. "You dance with them what brung you."

I started and was nearly to him when he shut up, but, as sometimes happens, he shut up one gobble too soon. I was maybe there and maybe not, not close enough to be certain, but way too close to do anything stupid like moving anymore until I was sure.

The proper move at this time is to stay where you are, sit down, stick to your blind, conduct yourself as if he were within a hundred and fifty yards, and play out the string all the way to the end. There is really no other intelligent choice, thin and flimsy as the choice may be at the time.

I did all that. After I sat down and waited until I was reasonably sure that any sensible turkey had probably flown down from the roost, I yelped one time.

There was no answer, no sound, no nothing.

Last year I bought one of those new seats that have come out recently. It has legs about three inches long, with the front legs somewhat longer than the back to give it a comfortable pitch, and a woven web seat like a lawn chair. It is a marvelous invention, but it has one defect. You can put it too far from the tree so that when you lean back against the trunk, you are uncomfortable. I had done that, so I carefully eased up, knelt down, and with my back to the blind, moved the seat a couple of inches closer to the tree.

Behind me, in the part of the world I should have had under observation, I heard a turkey fly.

Not fly away scared, not the two or three light flips of flying down, not the regular prolonged beat of flying up; just four or five regular flaps, like maybe he had flown across a slough.

Convinced that I had committed aggravated stupidity for the four thousandth time, I took several minutes to get turned around, sit back down, and get the gun up on the left knee, expecting every second to hear the sharp putt that means:

"Gotcha! You lose again."

Nothing happened at all, except that way down to the south, for no other reason than simply to rub it in, Old Faithful cranked up and began to gobble fit to choke himself.

Nailed now from both directions, crucified on the same cross of intellectual insufficiency I have carried for years, I sat quietly, conducting an inventory of my sins, when a turkey gobbled right in front of me.

And when I say right in front, I mean right in front. Right there. Right under my feet. So close I could hear the rattle in the bottom of it, so close it made me jump, so close the unexpectedness of it scared me a little, except for one thing.

There wasn't any turkey out there.

The area is a mixed stand of fifty-year-old pine and hardwood with a closed crown. It is nearly without understory, and the density of stocking is such that there is almost nothing larger than fourteen inches at the butt, and nothing that size was directly in front of me. There was nothing out there big enough to hide a turkey gobbler, except one who was standing behind a tree, stretched out three inches wide and six feet tall, like Wile E. Coyote in the "Roadrunner" cartoons.

Unless the turkey was invisible.

Or unless he, and I, and the whole southwest corner of Alabama had been moved through the looking glass and magically transported into another dimension.

Neither event had happened, but he let me sit there for almost five minutes, disoriented, with the hair on the back of my neck standing straight out like a Neanderthal attending his first eclipse, until he bothered to furnish an explanation.

Thirty yards in front of me was a twelve-inch pine. He dropped down out of this with his wings cupped, like a duck, not sailing but dropping almost straight down.

The wing noises I had heard were those he made when he landed in the tree, and there were enough branches up there to keep him from seeing me while I was turning back around. The fact that I had my back turned when he came had kept me from seeing him when he flew in.

Not only did it never occur to me to look up, it never even occurred to me to *think* up. I couldn't have seen him because of the branches anyway, and turkeys that gobble that close have never flown up to me. They have invariably walked up slowly. Usually very, very slowly.

You look up for geese; for turkeys, you look on the ground.

I didn't even try to shoot him.

We plain, simple people, who do not make a living as practicing witch doctors, handle the occult very poorly. Things like him, creatures playing in a higher league altogether, might even be ephemeral, "hants," things with an invisible force shield that can repel a charge of shot.

To tell you the truth, I was afraid to shoot him. It might have backfired.

He might have gotten angry and turned me into a frog.

Because there may even be a further dimension. There may be things that are so far over into H that they are nearly on the ragged edge of I.

16

Lonnie

PEOPLE WHO SPEND a great deal of time outdoors and who follow occupations that require walking in the woods a great deal always seem to age well. I do not refer to the practice of wearing those cute little walking shoes and shorts and restricting movement to cleared trails that have signposts to tell you how far you have come and how much farther there is to go before you get to the next shelter. My reference in this instance refers to walking cross-country. Walking cross-country here in the southeast, wearing nothing but walking shoes and shorts, would require a blood transfusion by ten o'clock on the first morning because your legs would not simply be scratched, they would be very nearly flayed.

People who cruise or mark timber will normally use up a pair of boots every six months, and sometimes, depending on the area, wear out three pairs a year. I have never worn out a pair of boot soles by walking. The vines and briars cut the tops off long before the soles wear out. Timber cruisers, whose profession requires them to travel in straight lines regardless of briar patches, would never have to tell people what they did for a living if they were members of nudist colonies. They would be the ones with the legs that looked as if they had been wading through cat fights, and these scratches are inflicted through a pair of work pants.

Off-trail walking while wearing shorts through the number

of things in our woods that have thorns, spines, or stickers is simply out of the question.

Woods work that consists mainly of walking to cruise or mark timber or look after woods operations of one kind or another constitutes light exercise. Logging, especially as it was done in the days before the advent of highly mechanized systems, was not only hard work, it was brutally hard work, and people who do that kind of work not only do not age well, they burn out early. Logging as done in the severe conditions of heat and humidity that exist down here on the edge of the tropics is debilitating even in mechanized logging operations, because even in mechanized operations there are usually some people on the ground.

There are now air-conditioned skidders and loaders. Log truck drivers run air-conditioned haul trucks, and crane operators at concentration yards sit in air-conditioned cabs.

Nobody yet has been able to devise a way to air condition a chainsaw, and anybody in a logging crew who does not ride equipment but works outside on the ground earns his bread by the sweat of his brow just like the Lord promised Adam he would do after that incident involving the snake and the apple.

Take an August afternoon with both the temperature and humidity between ninety-five and one hundred degrees with no wind. Put the logging crew near the edge of what is known in this country as a crawfish flat—which is a low, wet area filled with pitcher plants—and the man on the ground will find himself with a very sweaty brow indeed.

So will a timber cruiser, but timber cruisers were formerly armed only with a compass and a pencil, and modern timber cruisers nowadays carry nothing but a two-pound data recorder.

A saw hand operates a chainsaw, and it is not one of those light-weight models you see in the hands of suburban house holders playing with the firewood in the backyard. It is an industrial model chainsaw and comes out of the box with some heft to it.

Baseball players call the mask, the chest protector, and the shin guards worn by a catcher the tools of ignorance.

Running a chainsaw in a logging crew in August is an instance of the tools of ignorance cubed, rather than squared. Because operating a saw is the entry-level job in logging crews all across the South, the pay scale is substantially below that enjoyed by catchers in either the minor or the major leagues.

Arrangements can be made in rates of pay. Certain modifications can be made possible with working conditions and hours, but the job of saw hand remains very like that of an infantryman. The nature of the job itself creates the hazards that accompany the position.

And for the same physical reasons that catchers are gone from the roster at the age of forty, saw hands are worn out at fifty. Far more worn out than ex-catchers, as a matter of fact, and with nothing even remotely approaching a comparable state of financial position to fall back on.

There are far fewer professional, long-service saw hands than there used to be. Promotions to equipment operator or truck driver generally come from the ranks of saw hands, and as both these jobs pay better and sweat less, they encourage saw hands to be ambitious. But in small organizations there may be very few options, and even in large ones there are people with very little mechanical aptitude. These people tend to remain professional saw hands for years.

As they begin to get to the age at which they cannot keep up physically, it is usually possible to make arrangements, providing the operation is large enough and has a variety of things to do in other lines. What is required is that the organization recognize the problem and exercise some ingenuity in solving it.

Lonnie Barnes was a prime example of the very best type of professional saw hand.

He was not simply good at his job, he was excellent. He came early, he stayed late, and he took things personally. It was never necessary to oversee Lonnie; you simply told him what was necessary, then got out of the way to let him do the job. He frequently expanded upon his instructions in a manner that gave better results than if he had followed the originals verbatim.

But put him on a skidder and he was a disaster; let him try to operate the loader and you stood a first-class chance of having most of a log truck flattened by dropped logs; turn him loose on the public road with a truckload of logs and the lawsuits would have fallen not as does the gentle rain from heaven, but as did the deluge. Lonnie was a great saw hand, a lovely human being, and a splendid employee—with a power saw in his hand. With any other piece of equipment, he was pure klutz. As he came to the physical end of his working career, we were able to move him to the boats as a deck hand in the same pay grade, and he served on the river until the normal retirement age.

He pulled his weight and more until the day he finally retired, and the position we found for him on the river not only was a round peg in a matching hole for us, it fitted marvelously into his compulsive avocation.

Because Lonnie fished.

The three words have been put into a paragraph by themselves deliberately, because Lonnie's fishing was not simply something he did as a hobby. It was a separate part of his life. It was not only a separate but equal part, it was a separate and superior part in every respect.

As part of the river operations system, there was a deck barge with living quarters, its own small tug, a front-end loader, and a crane to load logs into hopper barges. This entity left the central docks on Monday morning, picked up wood cut and left on the river bank by a trap line of logging operations (to include the helicopter logging job), and loaded barges and left them tied to the bank for one of the line boats to gather up and carry south on its normal run.

Inspired to a degree by Damon Runyon's description of the oldest, permanently established, floating crap game in New York, this operation constituted the first, permanently established, floating wood yard on the Tombigbee River.

Living quarters on the deck barge were comfortable, sparkling new, and air-conditioned. The food was the best that money could buy, and if you ever took a look at the grocery bill, it would give you an idea of just how accurate that statement is. The only drawback to the duty station was the lack of night life and the paucity of feminine companionship. Between Monday morning and Friday night, the only official contact with the outside world was the passage of boats on the river, movies on the VCR, television, and the portable telephone. The best description for the location of the loader barge at the end of every day would have to be labeled as trackless wilderness.

There is an old saying current in Southern logging operations that "You may have to be poor and hired out, but you don't have to be stupid." In the paragraph above, you will notice that I have entered the qualifier "official contact."

Because boys will be boys and girls will help them; because

there were unlimited numbers of local phone calls made on portable phones from small boats and public and private landings up and down both rivers; and because there were willing hearts, there is no question in my mind that other, unofficial, private arrangements were sometimes made.

I have no idea of the nature and duration of these private arrangements. I never invented any reason to search them out. It is now and has always been my firm conviction that there are things going on all the time that are not the business of higher headquarters. Any private arrangements made by troops that does not affect the operation should remain the private business of those troops and needs no official recognition whatsoever.

One of the finest qualities of leadership is the capacity to recognize when it is expedient to smother your curiosity and let well enough alone.

As part of its on-deck equipment, the loader barge had a dinghy, complete with a small outboard motor. The barge parked every night somewhere along either bank of several hundred miles of river, and a compulsive fisherman whose time was mostly his own from the evening meal until breakfast the next morning could begin fishing somewhere in the neighborhood of a minute and a half after the dinghy was launched.

You may think that fishing five days a week ought to satisfy any normal man, and you may be right. But whoever said compulsives were normal? What Lonnie did every afternoon from the time he knocked off until dark was what is called in this country a "get by." Which means you can make do with it, if pressed, but it is only a barely acceptable substitute.

Turkey hunters who shoot doves in October before the turkey season opens understand get bys. Get bys are probably best described by saying they are analogous to the only game in town.

What Lonnie was was a redfish specialist, and redfish do not occur in the river systems much above the brackish water line. So no matter how much casual fishing Lonnie was able to do after supper five days a week, when the redfish were running in the early fall, he spent the weekends down in the brackish water, fishing.

Under normal circumstances, people who fish like Lonnie do not fish with people who fish like me. We make them uncomfortable in that we do not, in their opinion, take things as seriously as we should.

I consider myself to be guilty as charged.

When bream are on the bed, and two people will use up a hundred crickets in two hours, I go a little. From time to time, in sheer boredom, I will catch a few white perch on jigs and I have tried, because I read about it in Bartram, the scheme he describes for catching black bass on bobs, which works, by the way.

In the fall, when the redfish and speckled trout are running, I will try them just a little—until the dove season gets in the way. But by and large, I throw fishing into the same category as bowling. If you knock all the pins down, you get to knock them all down again—and who the hell cares anyway, except bowling alley owners and bowling league members in the Midwest?

People like Lonnie consider this to be heresy of the deepest dye, heresy as a matter of fact, teetering along the ragged edge of treason.

Lonnie and I crossed paths one October morning in the door of one of the fishing camps on the causeway where we had both stopped to buy bait. Lonnie was on his way to fish from the bridge over the Apalachee, and I had just launched the boat intending to run downstream to the marshy islands at the mouth of the river. Both of us were alone. I considered that prospects would be better down at the mouth rather than from the bridge, so I asked Lonnie if he would care to go along with me.

I remember telling him he needn't worry that any of his friends might see him in the boat with a fisherman of my class and quality because he could always say he was trying to teach me something, and he laughed, but it was one of those tentative laughs that demonstrated the fact that such thoughts of possible damage to his reputation had already crossed his mind.

Inherent politeness overpowered native caution, however, and he got in the boat.

At the mouth of the river we began to drift-fish live shrimp, without weights, downstream with the current. At the end of the drift, I would run the boat back up to the first island, and we would drift back down again.

The tide was falling, we had about a knot and a half of current, and there was time to have all sorts of conversations in between fish. Lonnie was catching two fish to my one, which left me more time than him to answer questions anyway, and we discussed wood flow, the state of the paper business, the possibility of expansion of the division, and the price of export logs, among other items of mutual interest.

I have long since gotten over being surprised at the depth and penetrating intelligence of some of the questions about the business that come from people who hold jobs well down in the rank structure. They read the same newspapers, look at the same television, are just as well informed, and just as able to have legitimate concerns as I am. The whole affair that morning turned into the relaxed give-and-take of a pair of loggers talking shop over the fish, until Lonnie quit being specific and turned general.

He asked me what caused the tide.

Questions about the job, the wood business, the possibilities of change in logging systems, the state of the art in logging equipment all depend upon a man's background and native intelligence. Understanding the tide, its dependence on the position of the moon and the sun, and the pull of gravity on the side of the earth away from the moon all require a background in elementary physics and astronomy that was not included in Lonnie's background in the kind of schools he went to for whatever length of time he was able to attend those schools.

I girded my intellectual loins, moistened my lips, and launched into the explanation. It was obvious that I had begun to lose him by the end of the first sentence. Things quickly went from bad to worse, and I knew matters were hopeless when the responses of agreement began to come before I had nearly gotten to the end of whatever point I was trying to make. The "Yes Sirs" were coming entirely too close together. At about the halfway mark—not halfway to a successful conclusion, but halfway to the point where it was obvious the failure was going to be complete—it became evident to me what was going on.

Lonnie thought I didn't know what caused the tides either, was too proud to admit it, and was simply creating a smoke screen of words to hide my ignorance while I bluffed my way toward an explanation.

I was not only the boss, but occupied a place several steps up the rank structure above him. He and I had known one another for years, had always dealt fairly with one another before, and he considered this to be simply one of those instances when one of a man's personal friends is showing his ass, and the graceful thing to do is to help him out of trouble and embarrass him as little as possible while you are about it.

Sort of like finding one of your friends falling down drunk and undertaking to quietly get him off the street and safely back home before he disgraces himself.

Good troops have the remarkable capacity to be patient with you when it is their opinion that you need help, and Lonnie did it as smoothly as I have ever seen it done.

At the first possible break point, he thanked me for the explanation, told me he had always wanted to know how the tide worked, gracefully changed the subject, and never showed by so much as the flicker of an eyelash that he considered every word I had uttered about the tides to be an unmitigated crock of shit.

I am inclined to doubt that the diplomatic service of the United States would ever accept any recommendation I might care to make. While it is not unusual for a recommendation for an award in the military to be made posthumously, it is not normal for a promotion in rank to be made after death, although there are such instances on record. The Confederate army, an organization that never awarded a medal during the whole of its corporate existence, promoted John Pelham after he was killed so that he could be buried as a lieutenant colonel.

In addition to the deficiencies of the nominator, the nominee would be deficient in several areas. Lonnie Barnes was not a graduate of Georgetown University or of any other seat of advanced learning for that matter. He is dead; his level of social polish could never be classified as glittering, and his written communication skills were definitely not of the first rank.

But in the fields of sensitivity, empathy, courtesy, and consideration, there is no person now in the diplomatic service who could in any way be his superior, and he is eminently deserving of a posthumous appointment.

Even dead, he is better than a lot of the live ones they have at home.

Soon as I get enough rank, I am going to tend to it.

17

Passing the Baton

ALMOST EVERY NEW PROJECT or process, especially one that involves a pronounced change in direction or procedure and requires a major effort, passes through five fairly distinct phases before completion. These are, in order of occurrence:

1. Boundless enthusiasm
2. Creeping doubt
3. The search for the guilty
4. Punishment of the innocent
5. Credit to the uninvolved

Phase one concerns itself with the first hot flush of creativity, the presentation of the project to the approving authority, and the bubbling public conviction that the thing is a sure winner. Initial proposals are invariably accompanied by reports and presentations that feature production rates or performance graphs shaped like hockey sticks and promises that these will require only the barest minimum of learning time before coming to complete fruition.

The implication is that the only unknown factor is the number of sacks that will be required to transport the resulting profits to the bank.

Phase two tends to develop in a gradual and insidious manner. There is no sudden dash of cold water, no financial Pearl Harbor as it were, but certain indicators begin to surface.

The possibility of delay is at least discussed. Revised performance curves are produced that show the slope of the hockey-stick-handle production-and-profit curves beginning to lean somewhat to the right. The time frames necessary for the completion of intermediate steps have a tendency to expand a little, and the existence of learning curves is alluded to for the first time.

In phase three, the extremely faint-hearted begin to look for candidates who can be blamed, and those who only suffer from a moderate case of panic begin to distance themselves from the project.

Neither of these two classes of faint hearts have totally abandoned hope, but both are uneasy. The scheme of maneuver of each group is to leave itself operating room to jump in either direction, depending on circumstances, but without making a visible commitment to any direction at this particular time.

Phase four absolutely turns into a total witch hunt in the event that the project appears to be failing. Conversely, some of the liveliest coat turning imaginable occurs when those things that appeared to be sliding down the tube miraculously recover. In the rare instances when a project has had few setbacks, little delay, and no apparent financial overruns, phase four can be almost undetectable.

It is always present, for there are always the faint hearts, but in successful projects, it usually stays under water.

Phase five is always highly visible and springs into full bloom irrespective of the outcome of the endeavor.

If the project is a howling success, people in higher headquarters who were barely aware of its existence gather in crowds to bask in reflected glory and assume wholly disproportionate slices of the credit. Here the innocent are punished, because those truly responsible for the success are ignored. In the case of failure, higher headquarters goes into a positive feeding frenzy. People in lower ranks who were not even consulted or concerned with the project are assigned segments of the blame. Many of them suffer disciplinary action for the results, and some are even terminated as punishment.

Major projects rarely conclude with a whimper, and the terminal bang can sometimes be cataclysmic.

A very closely analogous set of conditions comes into play

immediately after a person or a corporation acquires a new piece of equipment.

The boundlessly enthusiastic phase—complete with polishing, waxing, and showing off—lasts as long as the thing is still new and shiny. The onset of creeping doubt begins at about the time the new wears off or if it is discovered that there are improved models available.

There is no search for the guilty as such. This phase takes the form of a constantly growing list of inadequacies and inherent faults in the machine itself that have never been visible until now and, as time passes, these deficiencies become progressively more and more objectionable.

Conditions four and five are combined in the sense that the piece of equipment, having been found guilty of the crime of unsuitability because of length of service, is rationalized into a state of obsolescence and is punished by being replaced.

Aut inveniam viam aut faciam.

Nobody ever traded in a car or a house or a shotgun without, either consciously or unconsciously, going through something closely approaching these last steps. The single exception occurs when the piece of equipment has either been stolen or dropped overboard and has vanished altogether.

Such sloppy thinking is, unfortunately, one of the almost universal and wholly undesirable traits of human nature and, except for you and me, a common failing of us all.

It pains me to admit that even I was tempted, succumbed, and was guilty of exactly such a piece of self-delusion about ten years ago when I decided to change boats.

In my own defense—those of us who are guilty of any degree of candy-assed treachery always have a defense—the situation did change somewhat beyond the original set of circumstances that led to the creation and construction of the original boat.

To begin with, my home county elected to close the fall turkey season.

There was no biological reason for doing so. No game biologist I have ever known, who has any spark of intellectual honesty, has been able to give any biological reason for not hunting turkeys in the fall.

There are still about a dozen counties in the state that allow a fall season, although there are some that change and then backslide in one direction or another. I am convinced that clo-sure is founded on a combination of ignorance and laziness, and that the blame can be laid at the feet of deer hunters, all of whom possess both of the above characteristics in abundance.

Fall turkey hunting requires a great deal of walking. Until turkeys are found and scattered, the motion is not constant, but is nearly so. Now that deer hunters spend all of their time in shooting houses, some of which come equipped with magazines and rocking chairs (any day now I expect to hear of houses with wine cellars and adjacent putting greens for when things get slow), the idea that there may be people actually walking around in the woods at the same time deer hunters are sitting is found to be highly objectionable.

They feel it to be clearly within the range of possibility that such movement could inhibit the movement of deer to the green patch in front of the rocking chair, and this, obviously, cannot be allowed to happen. The safest course, therefore, is to forbid fall turkey hunting altogether. Many counties have done exactly that.

None of them, naturally, admit to this—the real reason. They have a mealymouthed list of specious, goody-two-shoes-type platitudes that they quote at length, like: "It is to preserve the hens," or "Too many jakes can be shot in the fall," or "Fall hunt-ing is too easy and is unfair to the poor little things"—all of which is believable to the kind of people who buy bridges with their life savings or who trade gold mine stocks with brokers who call from cellars in Montreal.

From where I usually launch the boat and get in the river, it is two miles upstream to get above the cutoff and hunt in Clarke County, which still has a fall season, and about that far down the river to a spot in Baldwin County, where I hunt the most ducks. Depending on the weather, clear and calm sends you to Clarke County, wet and windy to Baldwin. You have to make up your mind quickly at this launch and, in either event, you have to move rather briskly after you make it up.

While you are in no sense reminded of the spectator fleet at the beginning of the America's Cup trials, there is a good deal more barge traffic on the river than there was fifteen years ago. Upstream or down, you feel a sight more comfortable in the wake left by nine barge tows if you have more than fourteen inches of freeboard and ten mechanical horses on the transom of the boat, especially in the dark.

Not that the wake is any more severe in the dark, or the chop any more pronounced, but I have, unfortunately, gotten past the age that is convinced of its own immortality.

My luck, which I once felt was a block of ice the size of a bale of cotton, has been chipped down to no more than a medium-sized twenty pounder, about the size of the ones I used to carry home from the icehouse in my wagon.

Even after daylight nowadays, I am doing more travel by boat than formerly, going farther down the bay to fish, going over to the other river to visit, leaving aside the changing from county to county for various reasons. A little more speed is becoming more and more helpful.

And then there is the matter of weight. Thirty-five pounds is not a lot of weight. If you happen to be one of those Olympic Soviet weight lifters, it is probably beneath notice. Those guys probably wear thirty-five-pound wrist watches.

For wrinkled old men who drag boats around in the river swamp, and especially for those who have to drag one up the bank to get it out of the river and into a slough, the difference between seventy pounds and a hundred and four is a bunch, and every year it seems to get bunchier.

The answer to all these ills, for those of us with logical thought processes, of course, is to use two boats: one that is larger and more adequately powered for speed and one that is lighter, smaller, and handier that can be either towed behind the larger one or carried inside it.

Down at Head of Passes, the coon-ass duck hunters load two small pirogues aboard a hefty, beamy outboard with a lot of horsepower. They, of course, shoulder a cross we never have to carry over here on our half-size rivers: We have no wake from either ocean-going steamers or oil-field workboats to avoid.

Mouth of the Mississippi floating equipment, if used by duck hunters in our area, would constitute overkill in my judgment, but a degree of moderate downsizing would seem to be just about right. Maybe something of a somewhat smaller size, beam, and horsepower, towing one of the Staniels fiberglass duckboats I had seen at Head of Passes.

I tried just this, and it works great. In fact, once you get the length of the tow rope properly adjusted so that the pirogue rides properly in the wake of the larger boat, you can leave blinds and decoys in the pirogue and tow the whole thing back and forth to wherever you set up to make the hunt.

A Staniels boat could be reproduced in juniper just as well as in fiberglass, and if someone felt strongly enough, was a subscriber to *Wooden Boat,* and didn't want to be thrown out of the lodge, he could go that way just as easily.

But you drag the thing in and out of the river so much, you scrape the bottom so severely launching and recovering at concrete launch sites, and the boat spends way more time out of the water than it does in (which makes shrinkage and seam opening such a consideration), that it seems to me better to go with beaverproof fiberglass to begin with. Even us dinosaurs feel we are legitimately entitled to join the twentieth century now that we are just about to cross over into the twenty-first.

I admit this to myself now even though I would not accept it at the beginning of the rationalization exercises. At that point, I kept telling myself that the replacement for the boat would be made out of juniper and that I was only buying the thing in fiberglass because that was the only medium it could be bought in. As soon as I had the measurements and could gather up the lumber, I would begin the official replacement.

In the interests of expediency, and simply to keep things moving along while the new one was being built, I would use the new fiberglass model simply as a get by.

"Sure there is, Virginia. As a matter of fact, there are three of them, and four Easter bunnies."

Even while I was busily beating up on my conscience with a stick concerning the replacement and fooling absolutely no one at all with these half-assed evasions, one single thing kept sticking its head out from under the rug and refusing to stay swept under.

And that was the answer to the question of what was going to happen to the old boat.

You cannot take something you have built yourself, something you have owned and used for thirty years, and throw it on the garbage heap like an empty tin can.

A gun you no longer use can be oiled and racked along with every other weapon you own and committed to honorable retirement on the unused side of the gun cabinet. An old dog can be retired to a warm corner of the hearth and left to snooze in front of the fire until his time comes.

A boat is too big for a cabinet, takes up too much room to sit permanently in the yard, won't fit on the hearth, and, unless you have the thought processes of Henry VIII who replaced most of his wives either through divorce or beheading (Jane Seymour, you will remember, escaped inclusion in the list only by dying on her own), you are obliged to make reasonable arrangements for its disposal.

I do a great many things poorly, but way up at the top of the list is disposal. I do disposal worst of all.

I could have picked one of the oxbow lakes on the river and left the boat there on a permanent basis. You can leave one down there, and if you are careful to turn it upside down every time you get through fishing and never neglect to tie it to a tree, the current can't carry it off. If you happen to be blessed with a feckless and irresponsible temperament, you don't even need to go get it before the high water comes up in the winter. You just leave it under the flood water until the river goes back down in the spring and then go get it, turn it over, clean out the slime and mud that has been deposited in every crack and crevice by the flood, and press on.

This, to me, would be an acceptable solution if the object in question were a log raft made of rotten water oak tied together with bullis vines. But anybody who would do such a thing to something made of five-eighths-inch, clear juniper boards that had been in the family for thirty years would also be capable of throwing dog shit on his daughter's Easter dress when she was on her way to church.

I wouldn't want to know a man who was capable of doing such a thing, let alone be one.

Because I had rejected abandonment, was unwilling to consider sale, and would not consider leaving it along the back fence for the weeds to grow in front of and hide, the only recourse left was to give it away. Giveaways are always easier to say than they are to do for the principal reason that you tend to pay far too much attention to the character of the person to whom the gift is being made.

Once, years ago when we lived in a house way out in the mid-

dle of a tract of timber I managed, someone abandoned a preg-
nant, mixed-breed dog in our front yard. She whelped eight
puppies one Friday afternoon and was killed in the highway by a
passing car the following Tuesday morning.

When something like this happens, there are exactly two
choices.

You either go hunt up a croker sack and a ten-pound rock,
or you go to the drug store, buy several doll-sized bottles
equipped with nursing nipples, make a call to the veterinarian as
to the composition of formula, and play the cards you got.

If you play the hand, and I have done it—once—it relieves
you of any social obligations you may have considered pressing
before you looked at your cards.

What you do, on three-hour intervals for three weeks, is feed
puppies. You have no other duties. There is no room for either
other duties or outside social obligations.

We raised all eight, although it got a little sleepy there at the
last. We decided we could keep two, and then to our complete
surprise discovered that what turned out to be the hardest part
of the operation was making ourselves give away the other six.

These were mixed-breed dogs with absolutely no redeeming
characteristics whatsoever. There was no way to mistake any one
of them for a direct lineal descendant of Sirius of Gleam, and
there was not exactly a half-mile long line of prospective owners
clamoring to adopt a single dog.

In point of actual fact, all we had was one lonesome, highly
tentative applicant who waffled in a different direction every
time the matter came up and whom we finally rejected out of
hand on the grounds of indecisiveness.

In order to be considered for the ownership of one of these
dogs, it almost became a requirement that a candidate come
with letters of recommendation and a note from his preacher,
his doctor, and his banker certifying as to the condition of his
spiritual, physical, and financial health.

We finally placed all six dogs—one of them twice, as a matter
of fact, when the recipient sent him back—in spite of the artifi-
cial handicaps we erected for ourselves. I am of the unalterable
opinion, however, that it would be possible to marry off six ugly,
argumentative daughters without dowry in less time and with
less trouble.

I did not take applications for the prospective owner of the boat openly, preferring rather to act as judge and jury privately. But criteria for consideration were roughly the same as for the dogs, except that I may have lightened up somewhat on the financial requirements.

But every conclusion I reached, be it primary, secondary, or terminally, all ended with the same name.

Lonnie Barnes.

Lonnie needed a boat to keep him from fishing off bridges on weekends during the redfish season. Lonnie would not abandon the thing in the swamp for the floods to cover. Lonnie would appreciate it more and put it to better use than anybody I could think of. And from the standpoint of the boat itself, it would have more fish scales in its bottom in the next two or three years than it had had in all the other years of its life.

Because the State of Alabama licenses boats and requires that a bill of sale accompany one in order to change the title, I hunted up Lonnie, told him the arrangements, and wrote him a bill of sale, turning over ownership for one dollar and other valuable considerations.

There is a Celtic superstition that holds you cannot ever give a knife as a present because to do so cuts friendship. Anyone to whom you present a knife must, in return, give you a penny—as the sale price—to stave off the bad luck.

I am not at all sure this holds as true in the case of boats as it does in knives, but just to be safe, I gave Lonnie a dollar and had him give it back to me in return for the bill of sale.

We shook hands over the transaction, Lonnie hitched the trailer to the back of his pickup, pulled out of the yard, and I watched until he turned the corner at the end of the street.

From that day until now, I only saw the boat one more time.

I was around the bend in North Pass one Saturday morning the following November, when they went by on their way to the grass beds below the marshes at the mouth of Blakeley. The boat had a fresh coat of duckboat paint, there was a brand-new ten-horse Johnson bolted on the transom, and Lonnie was sitting in the middle of the back seat, rigging up a rod and steering the boat by shifting his weight.

Properly loaded and balanced, and with the tiller handle in the middle, the boat would make gentle turns in whichever direction you leaned, leaving both your hands free to tend to whatever business you had in the tackle box. I had known it could do that. I had just never seen it do it with anybody else.

Neither of them saw me, both of them looked great, and to go up and make myself known would have served no purpose and may have been construed as checking up. So I stayed where I was and after they passed turned upriver and left without looking back.

Lonnie isn't with us anymore, nor are the overwhelming majority of the donors, the cast of characters, the soldiers, the loggers, and the blacksmiths connected with the total operation.

I donated the boat in good faith. The business with the dollar was simply window dressing to propitiate unknown gods, and I am not dissatisfied with the present position. Given the same set of circumstances, I would make the same decision, and there is no call to go back and revisit the one made previously.

There are no regrets, but there is a single reservation.

I don't know where the boat is, or who owns it, or what he does with it, if anything. There is no one in Lonnie's family to ask. Not that it is now any of my business, even if there were; but all the same, I wish I knew.

It went from boards to boat under my hand, after all. There were a great many old friends connected with the project, and we were all together for a long, long time.

So even though it is no longer my concern, and I have no rights in the matter, the first eight notes of an old song cover the ground perfectly: "I wonder who's kissing her now?"